Praise for *An Accident*

"Lembi Buchanan single-handec won big time. Thousands of people living with disabilities are indebted to her. A fearless and tireless advocate, she succeeded where others have failed. This is a remarkable story by an even more remarkable woman demonstrating courage, strength and fortitude against a formidable foe. *An Accidental Advocate* is also a deeply poignant personal story, about the power of love when a marriage is threatened by an unforgiving mental illness, time and time again."

-Kimberley Hanson, CEO, HealthPartners

"*An Accidental Advocate* is a starkly honest and intimate memoir of the effects of bipolar disorder on marriage, family and friends... also a politically outspoken essay on fighting for fair tax treatment for Canadians living with mental health impairments and episodic disabilities. Lembi Buchanan skillfully weaves together these threads of advocacy in the personal and public domains and demonstrates an abiding faith in unconditional love and in a democratic politics of tenacious hope in resolving historic injustices."

-Michael J. Prince, Lansdowne Professor of Social Policy, University of Victoria
Author of *Struggling for Social Citizenship: Disabled Canadians, Income Security, and Prime Ministerial Eras*

"Lembi Buchanan's memoir brilliantly captures the unpredictable exhilarating highs and the disruptive lows that are the reality for people, like her husband Jim, who live with bipolar disorder. I know this well, as my father was diagnosed with manic depression when I was a young boy. For four decades, he and our family struggled with this debilitating disease long before the more modern medications like lithium were readily available. But, most of all for Canadians with disabilities, this is an important chronicle of how Lembi challenged the Canada Revenue Agency, by winning a landmark court case while prodding parliamentarians and finally, when that was not working, mobilizing a couple of dozen health charities to build the Coalition for Disability Tax Credit Reform. Lembi was the catalyst that brought us all together and kept us going."

-Max Beck, retired (former President & CEO at Easter Seals Canada)

1

"An Accidental Advocate is not only a tell-all book of an exasperating campaign to take on the Canadian government but also a genuine love story like no other. Lembi discovered early on that all is not fair in love and war. Stacked against all odds, she remained loyal to her husband Jim, despite the trials and tribulations of living with someone with a bipolar partner that threatened to sabotage their happiness. Chipping away at stigma, Lembi captivates her readers with honesty, humour and humility. This is a must read for everyone because mental illness has no boundaries and shows no discretion. Anyone can be affected at anytime."

-Marion Gibson, Program Manager, Mental Health Recovery Partners, Victoria
Author of *Unfaithful Mind*

"Lembi tells a remarkable story of love, heartbreak and resilience that leads her to become the 'accidental advocate' for those who are confronted with a family member faced with a mental health diagnosis. She is a masterful advocate whose actions are a searing indictment of the inner workings of our Canadian tax system and have contributed to reducing the stigma that comes with a mental health diagnosis. This book can provide a thoughtful guide for those in the disability community facing these barriers."

-Mary Lou Roder

"Thank you Lembi, for this honestly poignant and painfully true account of the challenges so many families face, when dealing with mental illness, and how they are affected by the bad decisions our Canadian government and insurance companies make to save money. As a mother of a son living with paranoid schizophrenia, this memoir has hit the mark on so many levels! Coping with a crippling disease, while fighting the CRA for fairness, is a story I know all too well."

-Brenda Hildebrand

"How do you live with a husband whose functioning is affected by bipolar disorder? Lembi Buchanan was faced with this situation and found a way - by loving him for who he is, by being ready to step in when problems arise and by working for better understanding and support for him and those in similar situations."

-Margaret Parlor, President, National ME/FM Action Network

2

"Lembi Buchanan is not just 'an accidental advocate,' she is a fierce, forceful, keen, and determined one. This is a poignant and honest portrayal of the difficulties that people with mental illness have when trying to access the Disability Tax Credit and how Canada Revenue Agency has taken advantage of the most vulnerable Canadians in our society, and continues to do so... Families struggling to get help for their loved ones living with a mental illness will find a comrade-in-arms... who has become 'the conscience of the mental health community.'"

-Christopher Laine Summerville, CEO, Schizophrenia Society of Canada

"Courageous. Determined. Knowledgeable. Insightful. Caring. These words are how I describe Lembi Buchanan, my friend and my guardian angel. *An Accidental Advocate* will keep you on the edge of your seat as you visit the full spectrum of human emotions. You will discover that it is not easy to love someone living with bipolar disorder and yet, Lembi's love for her husband never faulters. Her memoir is a must read for anyone who wishes to understand a complex illness such as bipolar disorder and its impact on loved ones. I met Lembi at a time in my life when I was overwhelmed by the CRA. When she heard what I was going through, she took over my file, fought on my behalf, and resolved years of systemic mismanagement by a government agency that preys on the vulnerable members of our society. She is a warrior in its purest form."

-Arlaine Bertrand

"Lembi Buchanan's captivating memoir *An Accidental Advocate* shows how 'Love is not enough,'" certainly not enough to defeat the ravages of a severe mental illness, such as mania and depression. While not always perfect in controlling the manifestations of bipolar disorder, she and her husband relied on the medical evidence that lithium therapy was essential in keeping Jim alive. Lembi counters the antipsychiatry movement that denies the existence of severe mental illness by sharing a love affair that has endured for more than 50 years because she and her husband chose science over unfounded theories that have no basis in medicine."

-John E. Gray, Psychologist (retired)
Lead author of *Canadian Mental Health Law and Policy, 2nd Edition*

An Accidental Advocate

Lembi Buchanan

Marci len —
As always —
fighting for
farmers
♡ *Lembi*

The Beresford Press

Library and Cataloguing-in-Publication Data

Buchanan, Lembi
An Accidental Advocate

Issued in print and electronic formats.
ISBN 978-1-7389476-2-1 (paperback)
ISBN 978-1-7389476-0-7 (ebook)

1. Buchanan, Lembi, 1946-Biography 2. Buchanan, James, 1945-Biography 3. Mental illness-manic-depressive illness-bipolar disorder- depression, schizophrenia. 4. Canadian government-Canada Revenue Agency-Disability Tax Credit. 5. Tax Court of Canada.

Classification: LCC RC516 .B844 2023 | DCC 616.895

To Jim, the love of my life, and
my extraordinary children Jonathan and Larissa.
And in loving memory of William (Bill) Buchanan,
Jim's father, who was always there, providing
support when I needed it the most.

Contents

Foreword

An Accidental Advocate is a remarkable chronicle of law reform. But, distilled to its essence, it is a love story.

Lembi Buchanan's memoir is the story of how one woman, endowed with an indomitable spirit, set out almost single-handedly to take on an obdurate bureaucracy. But what shines through is her unflinching commitment to a loved one, her husband Jim, who lives with bipolar disorder.

Lembi persuasively outlines how his mental disorder rose to the level of "disability" that should have provided the Buchanans with the right to tax relief under Canadian income tax law. The Canada Revenue Agency (CRA) defines the Disability Tax Credit (DTC) as "a non-refundable tax credit that helps people with impairments, or their supporting family member, reduce the amount of income tax they may have to pay." The DTC is intended to offset some of the extra costs related to the impairment. But for those like Mr. Buchanan, the uphill battle to get the federal government to the do the right thing has proven all but insurmountable.

There was no choice but to appeal to the Tax Court of Canada. Although Lembi has never had any legal training, she represented her husband and won. As incredulous as it sounds, the Attorney General for Canada requested a judicial review of a decision allowing people living with a severe mental illness to benefit from the tax credit. Not surprisingly, in a unanimous decision, the Federal Court of Appeal concurred with the ruling of the lower court, that it was an "obvious case."

Lembi was counting on her success to make a difference for others as well. She demonstrated exceptional leadership skills, recruiting senior executives from national charities as well as her former Member of Parliament, the Honourable Carolyn Bennett, and currently Minister of Mental Health and Addictions, in her fighting for fairness campaign. Together, with political support from all parties, major reforms were enacted by Parliament in 2005. When she recommended that creation of a Disability Advisory Committee, the former Minister of National Revenue John McCallum appointed her to the new committee. Despite it all, subsequent governments introduced restrictive guidelines, pushing back many of the important gains for thousands of Canadians from coast to coast.

When the Conservative Minister of Finance, the late Jim Flaherty, ushered in significant reform with the Registered Disability Savings Plan, he recognized the additional costs of disability that families were facing. Announced first in the budget of 2007, it was brought into force by 2008, lightning speed for federal tax reform. Then why was the DTC so difficult to reform?

I got to know Lembi in my capacity as the Member of Parliament for Victoria. My first assignment was serving as the National Revenue Critic the federal New Democratic Party. When she came into my office in January 2016, I was struck not just by her intelligence, but by her extraordinary focus on getting a just result. As a former law professor, I led Lembi into the arcane world of administrative law, discussing how discretionary decisions could be curbed either in court or through other mechanisms. We shared articles and she absorbed the information like a sponge. I saw firsthand her determination and zeal. Rather than seeking to reform the entire tax system (something that has never been done since the Carter Commission was appointed in 1962), she focused like a laser on how the DTC was failing Canadians with disabilities.

An Accidental Advocate illustrates how the CRA is a bureaucracy out of control, reluctant to make things right, once and for all. Despite all of her efforts, and the assurances from senior officials over the years, that all is well, I remain frustrated and flabbergasted that more still needs to be done to ensure fair treatment, especially for taxpayers living with mental impairments. There is no question that our tax system needs a major overhaul. In the meantime, Lembi has never lost her faith in our legal system and continues to campaign on behalf of those who have been unjustly denied the income supports to which they are entitled.

Lembi's memoir is a David and Goliath account of what a single, determined "accidental advocate" can achieve. While it is inspiring at that level, it is also a deeply personal story about the challenges of living with a person with bipolar disorder. Her love shines through as brightly as her tenacity. In spite of her own heartache dealing with the unpredictable and disabling effects of the illness, she remains loyal to her husband, regardless of the cost.

There is so much to be learned from Lembi's journey, that of an extraordinary woman who has refused to give up on her husband and others suffering with a mental disability. I commend this book to anyone interested in social justice, law reform and the power of love.

Murray Rankin

14

Author's Note

When I set out to advocate for fairness in tax treatment for Canadians with disabilities, there was every reason to be optimistic. Anyone with common sense surely could figure it all out and fix any problems in no time at all. How was I supposed to know that common sense and practical solutions do not prevail in government?

Instead, I would discover an obstructionist bureaucracy obsessed with balancing the budget, even when it meant denying a modest tax credit to the very people who need it the most. In order to achieve its goals, our government was systematically breaking the law and getting away with it. No wonder, previous efforts to reform the Disability Tax Credit (DTC) had failed.

I first went to Ottawa in 2001 and I returned again and again for 20 years, trying to resolve historic injustices. I never lost my sense of hope. What I did lose was my trust in a government acting in bad faith. As recorded during the debate in the House of Commons on November 19, 2002, Wendy Lill, the Member of Parliament from Dartmouth, Nova Scotia, railed against federal tax collectors for "shaking these people down because they are easy targets, too tired, too vulnerable, and too poor to hire lawyers to fight back."

Plain and simple, our society discriminates against people living with a mental illness. I would learn the hard truth early on in our relationship, when my husband Jim was first diagnosed with manic-depressive illness or manic depression, and more commonly known today as bipolar disorder. The fight for fair treatment meant ensuring access to the best medical care and reliable job security, and when that failed, private and public income support programs.

Over the years, I championed my husband's causes with the expectation that the landmark judicial ruling, in the Tax Court of Canada case, *Buchanan v. The Queen 2002* would benefit thousands of Canadians living with similar challenges. And yet, our federal government has continued to defy the courts by misrepresenting the legislation, making it increasingly difficult for people severely impaired in their mental functions to access the Disability Tax Credit (DTC).

Why? Are these individuals somehow less deserving than people living with physical impairments? I hope not.

Bipolar disorder is a dangerous and deadly disease when millions of neurotransmitters start firing out of sync, causing extreme mood swings affecting how people think, behave and function. This brain disease is a very complex biogenetic medical condition where heredity plays a major role in the lottery of life. Although advances in drug therapies and innovative treatments have made an important difference in the lives of people living with bipolar disorder, many continue to experience life-long disabling effects that meet the eligibility criteria as it is spelled out in the *Income Tax Act*.

When we met, Jim and I were two lonely people looking for love. Within days, we were deliriously happy, our emotions riding an incredible high that neither of us had ever experienced before. And yet, within weeks, without warning, the balloon burst, and we came crashing back down to Earth and with it, our dreams for the future.

Since then, I have found myself struggling on two fronts.

First of all, living with Jim is like riding a roller coaster, exciting but scary at the same time. The inability to navigate his unpredictable highs and lows often left me doubting my own instincts as a wife and mother to do the right thing. I was tired of feeling guilty for my role in Jim's extravagant spending habits. Not that I could have stopped him. At times, I was simply overwhelmed by the burden of a disease that repeatedly disrupted our lives as I struggled with my own fears, my anger and my sense of loss.

Right or wrong, I refused to give up on Jim.

Nor was I about to let the senior bureaucrats at the Canada Revenue Agency (CRA) wear me down. Despite the odds, I was determined to beat them at their own game by ensuring that they play by the rules.

While it needs to be noted that there are some very good people at the CRA, even in the collections department, who are knowledgeable and sympathetic, the old guard still rules the roost. Over the years, they have demonstrated the brutal lack of understanding and empathy for people living with a chronic and persistent mental illness. Despite important amendments to the *Income Tax Act* and some improvements to the application form, it has become more difficult, if not impossible, for people living with bipolar disorder to access the DTC without appealing their case to the Tax Court of Canada.

18

Part I

Against All Odds

Chapter One – The Scales of Justice

Toronto May 28, 2001

The hearing of one of the most important cases ever appealed to the Tax Court of Canada was about to begin. And I was a nervous wreck.

The stakes were enormous. A favourable ruling would have a significant financial benefit for thousands of Canadians with disabilities. All the more reason for the federal government to play hardball. Or so it seemed when I bumped into my husband's psychiatrist in the elevator.

What is he doing here? I wondered.

I had not been advised of any witnesses called by the Crown to support its position. But there he was, my husband's doctor, carrying a six-inch thick box of medical files, from The Centre for Addiction and Mental Health (CAMH), formerly The Clarke Institute of Psychiatry, where my husband had been hospitalized several times.

Should I have been informed? I had no idea. I was on my own since we couldn't afford to hire a lawyer to represent Jim. Besides, I wasn't very optimistic about our prospects. Right from the start, it became quite apparent that we faced a daunting, if not impossible task, taking on the federal government. After reviewing dozens of rulings, it was obvious that we were at the mercy of the judge's understanding of the complexities of a mental illness, such as bipolar disorder, and the burden of the disease, affecting Jim on a day-to-day basis.

I had been married to Jim for almost 30 years, so I should have known a thing or two about the impact of his illness on his mental functions. Of course, Jim would have failed the majority of questions on one of the forms sent to the doctor for further clarification, such as, "Can your patient make a simple purchase?" No problem at all. What about the Jaguar he bought on a whim a few years ago? Or booking a family holiday at Walt Disney World while occupying a bed in the psychiatric ward of the hospital?

I had the goods and I was quite prepared to prove that chronic and persistent mental illness was a legitimate disability as defined by the *Income Tax Act*; and therefore, Jim was eligible for the DTC.

Although I had no legal training, I did my best trying to look like a lawyer, wearing my black blazer, a white blouse and the only black skirt in my closet, with its tiny white polka dots. My dress code may not have mattered to anyone else. But it mattered to me. It gave me the confidence that I needed to assert myself in an unfamiliar setting, a court of law. After all, I had every right to be there. I was fighting for fairness and justice and that's all that mattered.

I was ready when the clerk called out "All rise," as Judge Diane Campbell walked through the door and took her place on the bench.

Taking on the feds

As long as I can remember, the CRA has been getting a bad rap. And deservedly so.

Given the severity of Jim's medical condition, we were not prepared for his reapplication for the DTC to be rejected. The fact that he had previously qualified for the tax credit from 1990 to 1995 was irrelevant. Although the decision took three years of reviews of medical documents to determine his eligibility, Jim was still asked to reapply for future years because mental disorders were considered to be "temporary" as if a miraculous recovery was just around the corner. The letter from the Canada Customs and Revenue Agency (CCRA), dated April 7, 1994, advised Jim that his appeal was successful, but he would have to start the onerous process all over again and file a new application form for 1996 and subsequent years. (Prior to December 2003, the CCRA was responsible for administering tax laws.)

In the meantime, the rules had changed. The eligibility criteria had become more restrictive for people like Jim, living with a severe mental illness, cheating thousands of people out of millions of dollars in tax relief.

When the eligibility criteria for the DTC was revised in the mid-1990s, physicians were no longer required to spend valuable time describing in detail the disabling effects of their patients' mental impairment. Instead, they just had to check either the "yes" or "no" box on the form. The determination of eligibility for the DTC was based on a single, simple question regarding mental functions that had no practical application, nor would it provide insight into something as complex as the workings of the human mind: "Is your patient able to think, perceive and remember?"

The government was making an assumption of fact that was not true, that people living with "a severe and prolonged mental impairment" were unable to think, perceive and remember. While the question may have been appropriate for an individual with a neurological disorder or brain injury, it excluded anyone diagnosed with mood disorders or schizophrenia. The question disregarded the intricacies of a serious mental illness since it did not address the likelihood that an individual's thought processes could be erratic, bizarre, deranged, dysfunctional or delusional. Not even a doctor's suicidal or homicidal patients could technically qualify if they had the mental capacity to carry out their actions.

Why? The government was promoting a false narrative that people living with a chronic, persistent mental illness were not as disabled as people living with physical impairments.

Why? Because it would cost too much.

I made numerous calls and wrote letters, but to no avail. In his response to my correspondence, the former Minister of Finance, the Honourable Paul Martin indicated that the disabling effects of Jim's bipolar disorder did not meet the same threshold of eligibility as physical impairments that were "much more severe."

In his letter dated September 13, 1999, Minister Martin was painfully blunt, providing the following explanation: "If eligibility for the DTC were broadened to include situations you have described as well as persons with severe disabilities, the federal cost would be much greater than the current $275 million."

23

The tax savings for Jim, when he previously qualified for the DTC, was approximately $700 each year, a substantial amount for us, but next to nothing for the government treasury. The federal government was balancing its budget on the backs of the disabled by its narrow and technical interpretation of the *Income Tax Act*.

The timing could not have been worse. There were plenty of challenges just dealing with the fluctuations in Jim's mood, varying in severity from week to week, month to month and year to year. The cruelest aspect of such an incapacitating disease was its unpredictable nature. The onset of acute mania could be triggered without warning, without Jim or anyone else being aware that he needed urgent medical intervention and possible hospitalization. Even relatively mild stressors might be sufficient to precipitate a major crisis, and set off a debilitating depressive episode. In other words, the roller coaster ride could start up at any time.

Our relationship had been strained for some time and I was trying to get my own life back on track. I just didn't have the will to put any more energy into the fight against such blatant neglect of the rights of the mentally ill. So far, my advocacy efforts to have Jim's DTC reinstated had failed. Nevertheless, Jim was obsessed with the belief that he was entitled to the tax credit and took matters into his own hands. Jim was like that, determined, persistent and unable to let go of his right to the DTC. On February 20, 2000, Jim filed his own Notice of Appeal with the Tax Court of Canada. "Regrettably I am a victim of the bureaucratic process..." he wrote. "In 1995, I qualified for the disability tax credit - a year later I didn't."

Of course, Jim was right. He was a victim of government shenanigans, preying on some of the most vulnerable members of our society, who could not afford to hire a lawyer to claim a relatively modest tax credit. And so it was that I became an "accidental advocate." If Jim was being discriminated against, there must be others, hundreds, if not thousands, who had nowhere else to turn. The odds were stacked against people, unjustly denied the DTC by a tax system too complicated and expensive for an ordinary person to challenge.

Of course, not everyone was willing to accept an arbitrary decision they disagreed with and subsequently filed suit against the CCRA, as described by the former Chief Justice, the late Honourable Donald G.H. Bowman, during a speech at the 20th Anniversary Symposium of the Tax Court of Canada in 2003:

Most of them are small cases in the informal procedure where individuals, unrepresented by a lawyer, ignorant of the tax law and of the court procedures, and armed only with a sense of indignation at the injustice that they perceive to have been wrought upon them by unfeeling, arrogant and rapacious tax gatherers, choose to take up arms against the awesome might of the government.

I also refused to stand by when a government agency refused to play by the rules. I simply couldn't understand the lengths that the CCRA would go to prevent Jim from accessing DTC when he had previously qualified after a rigorous review of his case. After all, there had been no change in his medical status.

Fortunately, I discovered that the Advocacy Resource Centre for the Handicapped (ARCH) in Toronto had a complete collection of DTC-related cases appealed to the tax court in its law library. There were several binders and it took me a week to read them all.

I kept getting more discouraged as I read the decisions in each appeal; it became apparent that I faced a formidable task taking on the federal government. I was horrified to learn that each assessment by the CCRA is presumed to be correct, even if it is wrong, containing an error or a defect. A conundrum to be sure. The burden of proof was mine alone. I had to quash an assessment that was presumed to be valid and binding. No wonder so few cases, less than one in a thousand rejections, ended up in court. After reviewing dozens of rulings, there was no simple formula to follow.

In *Lamothe v. Canada 1996*, Justice Bowman acknowledged that it had become more difficult to allow the DTC for the 57-year-old postman living with bipolar disorder because, "the tests have been narrowed even more drastically with the recent amendments." Just the same, he conceded that there are exceptions:

The Court is persuaded that Mr. Lamothe's problem so far exceeds normal limits that he falls within the narrow boundaries of this section (of the Income Tax Act)... I should also say something about the approach that this Court should take in these disability cases. They are small cases. To the taxpayer they mean a fair bit, and I've seen many of them and I can say that it breaks my heart to see the state some people are in and sometimes they just don't make out their case. But I think that is important that this Court bear in mind the very restrictive nature of section 118.4, and to the extent that we can, that we alleviate against that strictness and that we approach the matter with a degree of compassion and understanding that achieves the objective of this section.

In *Larivière v. Canada 1995*, Judge Murray A. Mogan took a different approach and dismissed Mrs. Lariviere's appeal altogether. Although she was unable to work due to the severity of her bipolar disorder, Mrs. Lariviere was still able to go out with her friends to play bingo and liked to watch television. In his ruling Judge Mogan wrote:

She played more than one card in each game; she followed the "caller" by marking the appropriate letter on each card. And she recognized when she had a winning combination of letters in one line. She watched television and identified certain favourite programs like "The Young and the Restless." She knew the characters in her favourite programs and was able to follow them from one episode to the next.

The confusing thing about a mental illness, regardless of severity, is that it never takes over a person entirely. Like many people who live with bipolar disorder, Jim could be very persuasive and convincing in his arguments when he was unwell and may have required hospitalization against his will. Jim also had the uncanny knack of masking the symptoms of his illness. He was able to hide behind a seemingly rationale façade while his manic mind may have been sharper than ever. And as far as Jim was concerned, he did not need someone to assist him with his financial affairs despite a track record of excessive spending that he could ill afford. We never knew at what point his judgment was distorted or flawed. We never knew when he was scheming to engage in inappropriate, irrational or harmful behaviour.

Still, I had to give Jim an enormous amount of credit. While I was filled with doubt, he always believed in his case, that he had a right to the DTC in the eyes of the law. Jim never doubted, not for a minute, that he would win this fight and asked me to represent him. Jim assured me that I would be successful; he became my biggest cheerleader, urging me to take the bold steps needed to right a wrong, not just for his sake, but also on behalf of thousands of others who were unjustly denied the DTC.

But first, we asked our adult children Jonathan and Larissa if they had any concerns, since the hearings were open to the public. Regardless of easy access to court documents providing the intimate details of their father's struggles with bipolar disorder, they were very supportive. As far as Jonathan and Larissa were concerned, a positive outcome could make a difference in the lives of other families as well, those with a parent or a child living with a mental illness, and that was nothing to be ashamed of.

Common sense and compassion

I appeared alone in court on Jim's behalf. I need not have worried about taking a chance by suggesting that he stay at home. Judge Diane Campbell accepted the fact that Jim was not present, noting the following in her ruling:

The Appellant did not testify and was not present at the hearing. His wife, Lembi Buchanan, who has power of attorney for her husband, testified. Given the evidence of Mrs. Buchanan, it is quite understandable why he was not in court. I believe the best evidence of his medical condition is from his wife who had the strength and fortitude to reside with this individual over a 30-year period.

I was barely out of the starting gate when Scott Simser, representing the Crown, objected. He argued that the historical record of Jim's illness and previous hospitalizations were irrelevant. Judge Campbell disagreed and advised me to continue.

There was no point arguing whether my husband had the capacity to "think, perceive and remember." Indeed, many of his activities required considerable skill in managing each of these attributes. I focused on Jim's state of mind when he was ill, and how the process of thinking, perceiving and remembering was dysfunctional, irrational, possibly psychotic, and sometimes, harmful.

I also spoke about the unpredictable nature of such an incapacitating illness. Individuals, such as Jim, who had already experienced several psychotic episodes, were always vulnerable to another relapse. I explained how Jim could be sane and insane simultaneously; how he could be in control and out of control, at the same time; and how he could be lucid, thinking clearly, and yet manic with thought processes on a much higher plane than the norm, as high as the heavens above. No one, not me, nor his children or his doctor might be aware that Jim was seriously ill, and might need to be hospitalized.

When it was all over, Mr. Simser asked to have the case dismissed altogether on a technicality.

"How can he do that?" I blurted out.

I couldn't believe that all my efforts preparing for the hearing could be quashed without so much as a whimper. Judge Campbell quickly intervened by explaining that Mr. Simser had expressed his position and now it was my turn.

As it turned out, Mr. Simser didn't have a solid case.

Jim's psychiatrist, Dr. Robert Cooke had been called as a witness for the Crown; he was expected to support the government's position that Jim was not markedly restricted in the essential survival skills required to function independently. Instead, his testimony underlined the complexity of bipolar disorder and reinforced my observations as noted by Judge Campbell:

The Appellant was "impaired by his illness" to the extent that he could not work, that he engaged in anti-social, inappropriate behaviour, experienced unpredictable periods of impaired judgment and impulsive decision-making based on his mental problems. He stated that in a number of areas, his ability to think and perceive is impaired. He indicated that he might be able to present well in public even when quite ill. That while being mentally impaired, he could otherwise function quite well at some level or perform some skill while the remaining thought processes were impaired… In fact, Dr. Cooke stated that it would be possible for the Appellant to be quite ill and yet even his own doctor would not necessarily recognize it.

In conclusion, Judge Campbell stated that she was "satisfied that the Appellant's impairment is severe enough to allow the credit." In a carefully crafted ruling, she provided an important summary of the dilemma that doctors are faced with when evaluating whether their patients meet the narrow and technical interpretation as far as the eligibility criteria for the DTC.

Although the Appellant is certainly able to operate adequately in some areas, his impairment permeates his entire existence. The facts support that while engaged in some seemingly rational activity to an outsider, all other thought processes are otherwise exploding in an array of erratic bizarre and potentially harmful activities. However, the Appellant's ability to perceive, think and remember, although not non-existent, is of such a severity that his entire life is affected to such a degree that he is unable to perform the necessary mental tasks required to live and function independently and competently in everyday life. I am convinced, from the facts presented, that without the constant supervision, care and support by Mrs. Buchanan, he would be unable to function on his own… I conclude that the Appellant's condition and resulting behaviour so far exceeds the normal and reasonable ambit that he comes within the otherwise very narrow confines of these sections of the Act… The facts quite clearly demonstrate that the Appellant does not engage in rational, logical, organized thought processes. His judgment does not permit him to function reasonably and independently. It is an obvious case.

Regrettably, it was not an "obvious case" for Jim's psychiatrist. Some might argue that the legislation itself was flawed. In her ruling, Judge Campbell addressed her concern that many physicians do not believe that people living with a severe mental illness are eligible for the DTC:

Dr. Cooke is quite obviously on a self-proclaimed mission to prevent patients getting a disability credit that, according to his interpretation of the Act, do not qualify for the credit. By bringing his own interpretation to these sections and his own preconceived notions of what activities might qualify, his completion of page 2 of the certificate was so coloured by his already formulated views in this area that I will not accept this certificate, as indicative of an independent, unbiased medical opinion. From the facts and evidence, it is clear, in answering the questions on the form, he clearly held the incorrect view that most individuals with mental impairments did not qualify for the credit... To go on to state in writing that most of his patients will not qualify for the credit... is clear and blatant bias.

I remember sitting in the court room, listening intently, but not quite understanding whether we had won. Not until it was almost all over, 30 minutes later, when Judge Campbell reprimanded the counsel for the Crown. She censured him not only for neglecting to keep me informed regarding concerns about the evidence to be presented in court but also misleading her:

I find the Respondent's counsel's attempt to hang the undertaking on the shoulders of the Appellant both reprehensible and misleading. At a minimum, I expect counsel to assume responsibility for that which he had not completed rather than deflect the blame on an unrepresented party.

Only then, did I feel a sense of vindication, listening to Judge Campbell's tough stance against those who conspired to deny the DTC to my husband. I was overwhelmed by a surge of emotions, the months of anxiety while preparing for the hearing with only a glimmer of hope that I might succeed; and finally, eternal gratitude for a judge who demonstrated that the court could find a way, as Justice Bowman noted in his ruling *Radage v. The Queen*, to interpret the provisions of the *Income Tax Act* "liberally, humanely and compassionately and not narrowly and technically."

Judicial review

Apparently, *Buchanan v. The Queen* was not an "obvious case" as far as the government was concerned. No doubt, the CCRA was concerned that Judge Campbell's decision could have wide-ranging consequences although cases heard under the Informal Procedure did not set a legal precedent. Still, other judges might consider the merits of decisions favouring the appellant and follow suit. In any case, the

CCRA was not about to take any chances. Within the month, the Attorney General of Canada filed a Notice of Application with the Federal Court of Appeal requesting a "judicial review" of Judge Campbell's ruling. The request was a clear indication that the government was not interested in fair treatment when determining the eligibility of individuals living with mental impairments.

Fortunately, the government was on the hook for our legal costs. As I was not a lawyer, I could no longer act on Jim's behalf in the higher court. The accompanying letter from Eric Noble, Senior Counsel for the Tax Law Services of the Department of Justice, advised him that "the Crown must pay the reasonable and proper costs of the taxpayer."

I was curious what might be "reasonable" and called Mr. Noble, asking him whether we were restricted to budget basement prices such as those offered at Walmart. Or, could we choose from top of the line at Holt Renfrew prices. Mr. Noble probably didn't have a clue of what I was talking about and declined to comment. As far as I was concerned, if Jim's case was important enough for the Minister of National Revenue to take notice, surely, he was entitled to the best legal minds that money could buy. After a few more calls, I was referred to Thorsteinssons, Canada's largest law firm specializing exclusively in tax law.

There was considerable interest in the case within the disability community. The Council of Canadians with Disabilities, the Canadian Mental Health Association and the Canadian Association for Community Living applied to the Federal Court for permission to provide oral submissions since the decision was expected to have an impact on thousands of Canadians with disabilities. A preliminary hearing for *Attorney General v. James W. Buchanan 2002* was held on April 30, 2002, with Bill Holder, counsel for ARCH representing the intervenors. Not surprisingly, the CCRA, known for its intimidating and bullying tactics, strongly opposed any intervention by other parties. Nevertheless, the Court was satisfied that there might be "public interest" in the case and granted the intervenors 15 minutes for their presentation. It was an important victory for our side.

On May 15, I was back in court but this time, I was not alone. There were plenty of familiar faces representing various health charities, an important display of the "public interest" in Jim's case. There was also an impressive roster of counsel, six in all, two for each party and two for the intervenors.

Of course, I was nervous. Jim's case was solid according to his lawyer Doug Mathew. But the Crown's counsel, Mr. Noble kept focusing on Jim's abilities, in an attempt to diminish the severity of his illness. After all, Dr. Cooke had testified that, "Jim could carry on a conversation, he was generally well-groomed, he could come to appointments, so he was not impaired in the most basic activities of daily living." In her ruling, Judge Campbell also acknowledged that Jim "is certainly able to operate adequately in some areas." However, she noted that Jim's "impairment permeates his entire existence... (and) is severe enough to allow the credit." Mr. Noble disregarded her assessment in his final remarks: "But your Worships, Mr. Buchanan drives a car. Surely that is an indication that he can think, perceive and remember."

Jim's ability to drive a car was never a matter of contention. Even at excessive speeds, while being chased by the police, Jim was a pro. Perhaps Mr. Noble missed the part in Judge Campbell's ruling that Jim "was able to cleverly and skilfully manoeuvre his rented vehicle... while being pursued by California police, all while under the belief that he was God about to receive an Academy Award... In other words, he can present himself as quite an intelligent, lucid individual while otherwise being in the midst of irrational and unpredictable behaviour."

In a unanimous decision, Justices Marshall E. Rothstein, Arthur J. Stone and J. Edgar Sexton dismissed the appeal. The ruling also established the legal precedent for the DTC for people living with a severe and prolonged mental impairment, including brain injuries, learning disabilities and Alzheimer's disease, who previously did not qualify for the DTC. We were subsequently relieved to learn that the CCRA decided "not to seek leave from the Supreme Court of Canada to appeal the above decision."

The date of the landmark judgment was May 31, 2002, my 56th birthday. Jim and I celebrated with a very fine bottle of Merlot from Duckhorn Vineyards in Napa Valley, one of the top wineries in California. Perhaps, with so many opportunities to celebrate, our relationship was fused together in a most unusual way. Even when there was nothing to cheer about, we still raised a glass of wine at dinner time, grateful for an enduring love that somehow continued to defy the odds.

It would be an easy bet that no one was popping a Champagne cork in Ottawa. The implications of the decision did not sit well with senior staff at the CCRA. Buried deep in Jim's file were two official responses for consideration, if there were any inquiries from the media:

The courts provide Canadians an independent review of cases and serve to clarify the law or resolve difference of opinion between the Canada Customs and Revenue Agency and our clients.

The Canada Customs and Revenue Agency and the Departments of Justice and Finance are reviewing the judgment to determine the impact.

First of all, there was no interest in clarifying the law to ensure a just result for others in similar circumstances. Secondly, there had to be an in-depth review of the consequences of the Federal Court's decision. In one of the most devious and deliberate moves so far, the government doubled down and conspired to tighten the screws even further. Within mere months, the CCRA introduced a new form designed to prevent Jim and many others living with mental illnesses from accessing the DTC, noting on its cover page that, "You do not qualify if the effects of the impairment are episodic or intermittent."

While unscrupulous insurance companies have been accused of bad faith actions, refusing to pay legitimate claims, our very own government was essentially following similar strategies by subverting the law as interpreted by our courts. And doctors were warned against bending the rules for their patients with the cautionary statement under the signature line: "It is a serious offence to make a false statement."

I was just getting started when launching my "Fighting for Fairness" campaign in 2001. I didn't know anything about advocating on behalf of others. I knew less about the political process. Surely, I thought, it would be easy to right a wrong. I was still naïve enough to believe that I could take on my archenemies and win. After all, I was not asking for special treatment; I was only asking for fairness.

I decided to capitalize on the interest demonstrated in my husband's court case and invited major national health charities and organizations to band together to lobby the federal government for fair tax treatment for people with disabilities. Jim suggested that I ask each of them to contribute financially to my work. He knew, better than anyone else, the hours of painstaking research involved with my efforts, and had a hunch that my life would quickly become more complicated. If anything, I could benefit from their expertise. Granted, the thought of financial support was appealing, but I worried that there might be some strings attached. My biggest fear was losing my independence. I still had some savings and decided to bankroll my own advocacy work.

My efforts on behalf of others drained my resources faster than my manic husband. I could not have anticipated how unscrupulous senior civil servants would become when challenged in the court of law. Nor could I have foreseen the relentless pushback by a government balancing its books by taking advantage of an entire class of disabled citizens, the mentally ill, those least likely to have the means to fight back.

How did I ever get here without a playbook of my own?

All it took was a chance encounter at an airport while waiting for a flight home for Christmas.

Part II

When Love is Not Enough

Chapter Two – A Match Made in Heaven

Flying high

Jim and I met 50 years ago, on December 22, 1972, at LaGuardia Airport in New York. It was standing room only as we were both waiting for the same flight to Toronto to spend Christmas with our families. No point arguing who was flirting, since I take full responsibility for walking up to Jim and starting a conversation. He was very good looking, dressed impeccably in a Bill Blass suit, peach coloured shirt and a nice matching silk tie. He was the same height and weight as me; even the colour of our hair was the same.

When our flights were delayed, we found a couple of seats in a crowded bar -- Chivas Regal for Jim and Jack Daniels for me. We were already a class act. When a snowstorm closed the airport, we lined up at Port Authority Terminal to board the Greyhound bus for the 12-hour overnight trip home.

Jim and I quickly discovered that we had a great deal in common. We had both married Americans a few years earlier and moved to New York. When our marriages failed, we stayed behind and tried to pick up the pieces. Although we became involved with other relationships, there were no long-term commitments. And then, within days, Jim and I knew we were destined for each other. We shared the same astrological sign, Gemini, with the promise of fun and excitement in the days ahead. Jim and I were both dedicated "foodies" with an appreciation for gourmet cuisine accompanied by fine wines. Unlikely as it may seem, our favourite restaurant was The Palm, a pricey steak and lobster house in mid-Manhattan that neither of us could afford. We were also passionate about art and photography and owned the same Pentax Spotmatic camera. Oddly enough, we had the same Crane's stationery packaged in a clear plastic box. As far as Jim was concerned, it was a sign. Were we a match made in heaven? We thought so.

Right from the beginning of our relationship, there was an easy intimacy with each other, a special magic, a certain chemistry, that happens, perhaps only once, in a lifetime and endures forever. Of course, we never questioned whether the euphoria we experienced was the real deal. As much as Jim and I wanted to believe that we were soulmates, our backgrounds could not have been more different.

Jim grew up in the exclusive Forest Hill neighbourhood of Toronto. His father, William Oliver Buchanan was a bank manager and his great-grandfather, James Oliver Buchanan was president of the Toronto Stock Exchange. His mother, Marion "Peggy" Buchanan, née Marshall, was a debutante with an active social life who attended finishing school in Switzerland. Although Jim, as well as his sister and brother, attended private schools, and lived a privileged life, he never felt that his parents were overindulgent nor did they play favourites. Whenever Jim was in psychological distress and required medical intervention, his parents were right there, always supporting him regardless of the circumstances.

I was born in Sweden. My parents, Vambola and Selma Pihel, née Lindstrom, both managed to escape Estonia when it was invaded and occupied by German and Russian troops during World War II. We arrived in Canada in December 1950 aboard the Cunard White Star *RMS Scythia*. I grew up in a working-class neighbourhood in the east end of Toronto, a few blocks from Woodbine Beach. My father was an electrician in the construction industry and my mother, who grew up on a farm outside of Tallinn, stayed home to raise five daughters.

I worked summer jobs and applied for student loans to put myself through university. Although I graduated with a Bachelor of Science degree from the University of Toronto, majoring in physics and biology, I had little knowledge about the complexities of the human mind that would, ultimately, turn our lives upside down. My research skills, along with the patience and perseverance required to manage laboratory projects, would serve me well when developing strategies to successfully advocate on behalf of people living with a mental illness.

When Jim and I met, I had never known anyone with a mental illness. Sure, there were stories of some college students experiencing "nervous breakdowns" before exams, but the colloquial designation was vague without referring to a specific medical condition. Even if I had some basic understanding of the ravages of a full-blown psychiatric disorder, I could not have anticipated the nightmare yet to come.

Especially not when New Year's Day was so perfect.

We were back in New York, walking in Central Park, holding hands and giddy with the excitement that we had found each other at a time when we both needed someone special in our lives. We were madly in love, and everything seemed possible and within our grasp.

Jim was the most charming, clever, captivating, interesting person I had ever met. His optimism, for our future together, knew no bounds. A marketing representative for the New York Telephone Company, Jim impressed me as someone who was not only very ambitious but also destined to succeed. His infectious enthusiasm for life was contagious. His magnetism drew me closer to him and it became impossible to let go. There was a seductive quality about his dreams for our future, to discover the joy of living life to the fullest which made me so vulnerable. He promised that we would each have our own Datsun 240-Z sports car and soon, there would also be children. My fate was sealed.

I was totally caught up with the euphoria that Jim was experiencing. How could I resist? How could I know that the seemingly perpetual state of "high" was caused by a chemical imbalance in his brain and that he was on a dangerous path to an acute manic episode?

I can't remember the first time I had a strange feeling, that it was all too good to be true, that perhaps Jim was not quite the person he was trying so hard to portray. It seems that Jim also had some doubts about our relationship in the early days with the following reference to his fears in a brief note to me:

To my love… I no longer have any fears in our relationship. I know it was meant to be. We are and were meant for each other. The excitement I feel is unbelievable. Nobody but a madman or a fool can comprehend what I feel…. My God, am I insane?

41

Jim believed in me and was certain that I was also destined for great things. Back then, I was a supervisor of Homemaker Services for the City of New York, working with families in crises and low-income senior citizens. Jim was impressed with my views on social justice and the need to improve living conditions for the people I served. He was a good listener as I shared some of the more difficult cases, which included fighting on behalf of my clients for better housing and good jobs. Nobody had ever treated me with such respect and reverence. I was shamelessly caught up by his attentiveness.

Jim could also be extraordinarily generous. He was delighted that I had a piano in my studio apartment and insisted on a mini concert. Although my rendition of Chopin's Military Polonaise was quite dreadful, he thought I had great promise. Later that week, he went shopping, spending more than $200 on sheet music and complete scores to a couple of musicals.

Our first date was an evening at The Metropolitan Opera to see *Madama Butterfly*. In Puccini's tragic love story, a young Japanese girl marries for love, but she is abandoned by the American naval officer based in Nagasaki when he returns home to the United States. I was mesmerized by the fabulous music and staging. Over the years, Jim would surprise me, again and again, with tickets to *Madama Butterfly* when it was performed in San Francisco, Seattle, Victoria, Toronto, Paris, and again, in New York.

Jim was also passionate about the theatre and well-versed in the Broadway scene. Even before we met, he had seen dozens of musicals and already had a significant collection of *Playbills*. Jim saw his first Broadway show, *Fiorello* about Mayor LaGuardia of New York when he was 15, while visiting his godfather who lived in the borough of Queens. When Jim was 18, he invested $1,000 in *The Student Gypsy, or, The Prince of Liederkranz*, a spoof set in the late 19th century in the kingdom of Singspielia. With great expectations, he flew down to New York with his friend Eric for the opening night performance and celebration for the cast and crew afterwards at Sardi's on September 30, 1963. Although the musical closed less than two weeks later, it has received rave reviews on the revival circuit.

In 1969, Jim worked as a press representative in summer theatre in New England. The theatre closed in October and Jim was back in Toronto when he applied for a position with a prestigious public relations firm in New York. The response to his query was not very encouraging:

Mr. Buchanan:

Before it is too late, please let me advise you to stay in Canada. You are greatly mistaken if you think that the world of theatrical publicity is anything more than drudgery, hard work, low pay and insecurity. What is more, the theatre in the United States is dying...

Were I a Canadian, I would apply for a position in the public relations staff of Prime Minister Pierre Trudeau. That, to me, would be stimulating and productive and you, no doubt, would meet a better class of people.

In any case, Jim was intent on pursuing his dream and managed to get a job as a mail room clerk with the William Morris Agency in New York. He was immediately assigned to the special services department, responsible for picking up theatre tickets for clients and escorting them to various venues in the city. Although it meant hobnobbing with high-profile celebrities, the pay was dismal at $70 per week. As an agent trainee six months later, Jim was only making $94 a week, not enough considering the lifestyle that he aspired to achieve.

With Jim's knowledge of the inner workings of the theatre, it was hardly surprising that he was able to get front row, house seats set aside for reviewers, for the sold-out preview of an off-off Broadway production of *The Hot l Baltimore.* The play was set in the lobby of a seedy residential hotel where the "e" was missing in its neon sign. As we waited for the show to begin, Jim pulled out a notebook and his Mont Blanc fountain pen from his pocket, and started to make copious notes. Afterwards, Jim thought nothing of crashing the backstage party. While I felt awkward because I didn't know anyone, it was clear that Jim was in his element. He became very animated when talking to the author, Lanford Wilson, telling him that his play would be a huge success. How could he be so sure?

And yet, Jim was right on the money. *The Hot l Baltimore* moved from the second-floor loft of the Circle Theater Company to off-Broadway where it won several awards including the New York Drama Critic's Circle Award for the best American play. A few years later, Norman Lear adapted the play into a sitcom on ABC-TV. I would experience the same uncanny insight and intuition, time and time again, as a public relations professional, throughout Jim's career.

We also went to see another play by Lanford Wilson, *Lemon Sky*, at a local church hall where we sat at a table with a bottle of wine between us. I don't remember the story, but I did record in my journal that Jim was very excited, convinced that *Lemon Sky* also had merit.

After the show, Jim was talking to the producers about possibly taking the play to Broadway. They were thrilled, believing Jim to be quite sincere. I was astonished by his brazen offer, but I should probably have known better, after seeing *Pippin* earlier that week.

Opening in October 1972, the musical comedy quickly became one of the most popular shows on Broadway. Jim had already seen *Pippin* twice, and agreed with critics that the frivolous medieval tale about the son of Charlemagne was a fabulous spectacle of magic and mystery. His only complaint was John Rubinstein's portrayal of the lead as he noted in this excerpt of a personal review of the show:

JR is a very good-looking boy with a lot of charm but lacks the depth of character that exists in the roles of the other actors... a blending of love of life, sexuality and everything else that makes it the brilliant musical that it is. The greatest show of all time... a total celebration of life, joy and love for man... that is so needed in this crazy world at the moment... Yes, JR is good, but he is not great. And Pippin is a great musical. Pippin needs a great Pippin – ME.

I found it hard to believe that Jim was serious about taking over the lead role, considering his stage appearances were limited to school choirs. The fact that he couldn't read music was irrelevant. He took out his notebook and wrote a memo to call the producer, Stuart Ostrow about the part. And he did so the following day, leaving a recorded message. Not surprisingly, his call was not returned.

Personal memos were becoming increasingly important to Jim as he tried to keep his daily activities organized. But it was becoming a futile exercise as his life was starting to unravel. There were times when he appeared to be completely in control. His fingers literally flew over the typewriter keys during a very constructive creative writing period. How could think that fast, let alone type at that speed?

The frenzied pace of activities after work and on the weekends drained me mentally and physically while Jim continued to have incredible reserves of energy. He also stayed up late, sorting through his papers and writing more memos. How could that be? I wondered. There were no brakes and there was no slowing him down either.

One day, after work, I told Jim I desperately needed a decent night's sleep.

"Tomorrow," he promised. "I managed to get really good orchestra seats for tonight's performance of *Jesus Christ Superstar*."

I hated the thought of wasting an expensive theatre ticket so, reluctantly, I agreed to go.

Despite an irreverent portrayal of the head of the Christian church during the last week of his life, the Broadway show was a huge success. While sitting beside Jim in the theatre, I had the sense that he could relate to the lyrics and music far more than I could. It was as if Jim was right there on the stage with the performers living through the agonizing betrayal of the son of God by Judas Iscariot. When the curtain call was over, Jim came back down to Earth. The association with Jesus Christ was already part of his DNA. I just didn't know it at the time.

One evening, we met two of Jim's friends from the office, Liz and Glenna, for dinner. They confided in me, saying how happy they were, to see Jim so energetic and engaged in a new relationship with someone he adored. Apparently, Jim had been quite depressed for some time when his first wife Brenda walked out on him more than a year ago.

Later that evening, I shared my own story with Jim, how I was in bad shape when my husband left me for another woman. Although I went to work every day, I dreaded going home to an empty apartment. Jim explained how he, too, somehow managed to carry out his day-to-day duties on the job but fell apart when he was home alone.

We had only known each other less than two weeks, when Jim moved into my apartment. Somehow, on his own, he loaded up a small rental truck with his belongings, including a full-sized dining room table, six chairs, a Sony Trinitron colour TV, and numerous boxes of vinyl records. When Jim mentioned that he was concerned that the Mafia might be following him, I laughed. I told him how my ex-husband threatened to send the Mafia after me if I did not consent to his terms in our divorce agreement. After all, this was New York, and the Mafia could be anywhere.

If Jim was experiencing paranoid symptoms, I wasn't aware of them. Instead, Jim was consumed with plans for our future and preoccupied with making more money. However, as soon as he started talking about quitting his current job to look for a company that recognized his true management potential, I became alarmed and expressed my concerns.

Jim assured me that there was no need to worry, trying to convince me that he could accomplish anything he wanted. As far as he was concerned, the sky's the limit. He talked about his dreams of producing his own musical based on Hugh MacLellan's popular novel, *Barometer Rising*, about the explosion in Halifax harbour during World War I. "Trust me," he said, promising to take care of everything.

In a well-organized resumé addressed to the president of a major insurance company, there were no clues to suggest that Jim's judgment was impaired. His statement about his goals, however, may have been viewed as being overly exuberant: "To want the best of everything. Idealistic, yes, but possible. I have the great need to experience life to the fullest."

On the other hand, Jim's neatly typed resignation letter to his employer, "Ma Bell," was a classic example of the manic mind. Although he was still very much in control of his thoughts, Jim's obsession with his self-worth was evident in the cracks of the psyche of an individual who was living in a different reality unknown to the rest of us:

It is with some regret that I write this letter of resignation... The fact is that for one and one-half years I have put the concentrated effort into my job without any just compensation beyond my weekly pay cheque and a few niceties from management... The name of the game in New York City is money. Money talks. The niceties are not enough... Strike three has long since been thrown. The ball game is over – "fini." New York Telephone's loss is somebody else's gain.

If only it were so.

I can't recall when our "perfect" life started to unravel. At times, Jim was irritable, even hostile, for no obvious reason. When I expressed concerns about his increasingly erratic behaviour, he assured me that he was "fine," that, in fact, he had "never felt better." Jim described his upbeat mood in the following note I later found among his papers:

I am on a most natural high that has no limits to its possibilities... the natural trips are fantastic. I decided last weekend that I was going to risk everything for a particular woman and I have and it has worked. No doubt about it. Yes, I am theatrical about (it), but all great men have to be. Yes, I am on a fantastic ego trip. But we must remember, so is a woman – a real wonderful person with a heart and honesty that cannot be compared. Our love will last forever. It is perfection.

The emotional roller coaster had been revving up for days, speeding faster and faster, making it impossible for me to jump off, even when there were some lingering doubts about a long-term relationship. I was brazenly caught up with the excitement Jim was experiencing and began to believe that it was all possible. Perhaps I should have known better than to trust him, but I didn't know that he was manic and his judgment, was severely impaired.

I discovered, soon enough, that it was impossible keeping up with Jim, and I often went to bed in a state of exhaustion. I also found it increasingly difficult to adjust to his shifting moods; and if I didn't agree with him, Jim became very agitated and dismissive of my concerns. I began to question whether we were really meant for each other, especially when we were fighting about money. I was furious when I found out that Jim had sent his letter of resignation to his boss without discussing it with me first. However, I wasn't prepared to walk out on Jim, not when he was confident that he would find another, better paying job soon.

Despite my apprehensions, I still believed that we would be able to resolve our differences. After all, most of the time, Jim seemed to be a reasonable person. He was also extremely resourceful, and I had every confidence that Jim would find a position more suited to his interests and abilities. We still had our hopes and dreams.

I might have been more concerned about our future if I knew about Jim's spiralling out of control credit card debt, now that he was also out of a job.

Sightings of the Secret Service

On a Monday morning, in early February, and unknown to me, Jim rented a car from Hertz and drove to New Jersey. I learned later that he was searching for the CIA. Although I hadn't heard from Jim all day, I only began to worry about his whereabouts when he didn't come home for dinner.

There were no red flags that anything was amiss, and there was no one to call to check up on him. I was relieved when the phone finally rang shortly after 10:00 pm. Jim explained that he had gone to see the opera, *The Masked Ball* by Verdi, and was on his way to a private party at the Lincoln Center, without providing any details, except to say that the Kennedys might be there. He suggested that I wear something sexy and meet him in half an hour. When I tried asking questions, Jim wasn't paying attention to me. Instead, he was racing through the events of the day.

Was I aware that President Nixon was in town? Apparently, his limo, parked near the Pan Am building on 42nd street, was surrounded by the Secret Service. Then, suddenly, Jim said he had to go and hung up the phone.

I got dressed, grabbed a cab on Second Avenue and headed over to the West Side, travelling through Central Park. When I arrived at the Lincoln Center, the plaza was empty. I found a security guard, but he wasn't aware of a private party on the premises. I checked the Ginger Man, a favourite Irish pub of ours, just across the street, but Jim wasn't there either.

I was confused as I walked back and forth along the sidewalk in front of the restaurant trying to make sense of Jim's urgent phone call. Surely, he would come looking for me. But 15 minutes later, I gave up, found a cab and headed back home. I was getting undressed for bed when the phone rang again. Jim was calling from the bar at the Ginger Man, asking me to come right over.

"Where were you?" I wanted to know.

Jim ignored my question. When I asked him about the party, he promised to explain everything. I reminded Jim that it was late and I was exhausted. Besides, the anticipation of attending an important party and the disappointment of not finding him anywhere was just too much. But Jim wasn't listening. Despite my protests, he pleaded with me to come. I was afraid to say, "no" because there had already been some angry outbursts on the weekend.

It was almost midnight when the cab dropped me off at the Ginger Man. Although the restaurant was still packed, I was relieved to find Jim sitting at a corner table. He smiled as soon as he saw me, got up and pulled out the chair for me. Jim was very charming, catching me off guard as he assured me that everything was fine. Rather than answering my questions about his earlier call, Jim talked about his "incredible evening." Apparently, no one stopped him when he wandered from level to level, watching the opera from various angles. "It was very exciting," he later wrote in his notebook. "I had some great visionary plans of my own. I felt a rush, a real high."

A waiter brought over an appetizer, *Coquilles Saint-Jacques*, Jim had ordered before I arrived. Without bothering to ask if it was OK, I casually picked up one of the scallops and popped it into my mouth. Suddenly, without warning, Jim's mood darkened. "How dare you take something that belongs to me?" There were other nasty words as well.

I was stunned not only by his angry outburst but also the verbal abuse. I had never seen Jim like this. For the most part he was a very gentle, sensitive, caring person who would not hurt a fly. Now, Jim was making a scene and I got up to leave. His sudden shift in mood frightened me. But he grabbed my hand, quickly apologized, and insisted that I stay. I didn't want to make matters worse, so I sat down again, and quietly ate my dinner when it was served.

It was very late when we finally left the restaurant. Jim had forgotten that he had a rental car parked underground across the street at the Lincoln Center so he called for a taxi to take us home. During the cab ride back to the apartment, I must have said something to provoke Jim because he told me to "shut up" and slapped me across the face. I was horrified by the sudden change in his temperament. I was also speechless, and it was just as well because Jim was oblivious to my concerns.

When the cab dropped us off in front of our building, Jim refused to come inside. Desperate to find out what was wrong, I followed him down the street. Rather than explaining his actions, Jim was threatening to leave me. He bragged about big plans for the future and his need to be in control. He was afraid that I would only get in his way. I tried to assure Jim that I loved him and would support him in all his endeavours, but he wasn't listening as he raced ahead of me. It was after 2:00 am when I finally crawled into an empty bed and cried myself to sleep.

I heard Jim come home a few hours later. He walked over to the bed and held me close. Jim was remorseful, with tears in his eyes, telling me how sorry he was and how much he loved me. He also assured me that there was no reason for me to be fearful about our future and soon enough, I fell asleep in his arms.

When I woke up, Jim was dressed, wearing a well-worn pair of jeans and a casual shirt. He was busy packing some personal items and papers along with a few notebooks into a box, as if he was moving out after all. I asked Jim what he was up to and started to get out of bed to make coffee.

Suddenly, Jim was on top of me, beating me with his bare hands. I shouted at him to stop and just as abruptly, he stopped, promising not to hit me anymore, if I stayed in bed. I'll never forget the distant look on his face. I was terrified, lying there in a state of shock. One day, Jim was deliriously happy about our relationship telling me that I was the best thing that ever happened to him. The next day, he was suspicious of my motives, angry and threatening. Without warning, Jim violently assaulted me for no reason at all. At least, that's what I thought.

It seemed to take forever for Jim to get organized as I lay trembling under the covers. Then, after grabbing the box and his elk fur jacket, he was gone. Jim also took my keys and locked me inside, so I couldn't follow him. We were living in a ground floor garden apartment with a security lock that also required a key to open the door from the inside, if it was locked from the outside.

I learned several weeks later that Jim had been listening to secret codes and messages over the radio, night after night, when I was asleep. The auditory hallucinations were very real, sending him on an important mission to save the world. He simply could not afford to take any chances, that I might try to stop him.

I was terrified that Jim might return, so I called Laurie, who lived nearby and asked if I could spend the day at her apartment. She and her husband, Spencer were among my best friends. I already had a set of their keys so I could feed their pet squirrel, when they were away on weekends. They weren't interested in having children and a dog would be too much trouble, so one day, they brought home a squirrel from Central Park. He wasn't a good pet, but they were crazy about him. I managed to "escape" out the back door that opened to our yard though, I had to climb over several fences before I reached the street.

All of the dreams Jim and I shared had evaporated like a mirage in the desert. My life was in shambles. I was confused and hurt. I couldn't understand how this wonderful person who I fell in love with could suddenly turn out to be such a monster. Of course, I wasn't aware that Jim had been exhibiting classic symptoms of bipolar disorder, almost from the day we met.

It was dark outside when Spencer and I walked over to my apartment to meet the locksmith. The police had also been notified. While the lock was being replaced, the policeman took out his notebook and wrote down some of the details as I went over the events of the morning. He commented on the bruises on my face and asked if I wanted to press charges.

"No," I responded without any hesitation.

My voice was barely above a whisper. I didn't want to have anything to do with Jim anymore. I certainly didn't want to see him again. Like so many women who have been abused by their boyfriends and husbands, I just wanted the nightmare to end.

No sooner had the policeman left when the phone rang.

"Mrs. Buchanan?"

Who would be calling? I wanted to say that there was no "Mrs. Buchanan" and hang up the phone. But Jim had already told his friends that we would be getting married soon and perhaps someone was just trying to be cute. On a far more serious note, the caller identified herself as an ER nurse at Metropolitan Hospital.

"Your husband," she explained, "was brought here by the police. We need to have you come and sign some papers so he can be admitted."

I didn't understand why Jim was being hospitalized if the police were involved. The nurse had been reluctant to provide further details over the phone. For all I knew, Jim had been injured in an accident and required medical attention. I grabbed my purse and rushed to the hospital.

I found Jim in the corner of the ER with two police officers sitting behind him. His jeans were torn. His shirt was dirty. Jim was wearing someone else's shoes that were far too big for his feet. There was a vulnerability about him that caught me by surprise.

"Hi!" said Jim, when he saw me. He was smiling as if he didn't have a care in the world, the very same irresistible smile that I was drawn to while waiting for our flight home to Toronto. The admitting nurse at the desk was busy so I sat down beside Jim, as he reached over and touched my face gently, asking if it hurt. Incredible as it may seem, Jim was unaware that he had caused the injuries. Then he lowered his voice and whispered, "The Mafia was after me again. So, I'm lucky to have police protection. They know all about my mission and are here to look after me."

I soon learned that Jim had managed to climb up to the roof of St. Patrick's Cathedral where, apparently, he was waiting for a helicopter to take him to God. Some workmen managed to guide him back downstairs where the police were waiting for him. It was obvious that Jim was delusional and needed to be hospitalized. As upset as I was with Jim, I was still hesitant about leaving him in a public city hospital with limited resources. A friend of mine had talked about the excellent care she had received at Payne Whitney Psychiatric Clinic, a private facility affiliated with Cornell University and New York Hospital.

I asked to use the phone while Jim was still in the ER with the police sitting behind him. When I was connected with Dr. Andrew Smithers, a resident doctor at Payne Whitney, I shared the information from the admitting nurse. I also tried to recount some of Jim's symptoms, the racing thoughts, ambitious plans, grandiose delusions and sleepless nights as well his volatile mood. Dr. Smithers explained that in all likelihood, Jim suffered from manic-depressive illness. He indicated an interest in having Jim as a patient because Payne Whitney was conducting clinical trials with lithium, a promising new drug therapy that was revolutionizing the treatment of this mysterious brain disease. I was relieved to learn that there was a diagnosis for the bizarre and outrageous behaviour I had been witnessing during the past month. I was also hopeful that a successful medication regimen might give Jim and me another chance at happiness.

The only hitch was that a bed would not be available for a few days and that Jim would still need to be hospitalized in a secure psychiatric ward. Considering the delusions Jim was experiencing, I was advised that he would probably be heavily sedated in the interim. Dr. Smithers also explained that it would be important for Jim to sign the paperwork needed to admit himself as a voluntary patient so that there would be no issues when it came time to transfer him to Payne Whitney. He was also very adamant about transferring Jim by ambulance rather than a cab because he could be a flight risk.

I don't know if Jim understood anything about the plans to move him to another facility in a few days, but he was willing to sign the admission papers in the interim. When an orderly came to take Jim to the psychiatric ward, I wondered, How could I have been so wrong about him?

By the time a cab dropped me off at home, I was exhausted physically and emotionally. And I had never felt so alone. I opened the bottle of Jack Daniel's, poured myself a stiff drink, and called Jim's father.

Déjà vu

Jim's father listened patiently as I relayed the events of the last few days while trying to explain why his son had been hospitalized. There was a long pause before he responded. "Jim has a long history of mental illness," he explained. "So it's not the first time he has been hospitalized in a psychiatric ward. We were so hopeful when he met you and we all thought, 'Thank God, he has finally met someone who will provide some meaning and stability in his life.'"

I mentioned the possibility of having Jim transferred to Payne Whitney. I knew nothing about Jim's medical coverage from his former employer or the state of his personal finances. His father's response would be repeated time and time again, whenever Jim ended up in the hospital, leaving me to pick up the pieces: "We'll do everything we can." He asked me to book him into a reasonably priced hotel in our neighbourhood for an indefinite stay; he also let me know that he would catch a flight to New York the following day.

I poured myself another drink. But there was no one else to call. What would my friends say? Not surprisingly, Laurie had suggested that I should "dump him" because he was abusive, both verbally and physically.

I certainly couldn't call my own parents. I had never been able to rely on them for emotional support, certainly not when my first marriage failed. My mother wrongly blamed me for causing a "scandal" within her own universe of a strict Baptist congregation. Instead of offering some words of comfort, she essentially ostracized me, as if I had committed a heinous act. As far as she was concerned, I was a failure, and an embarrassment to her.

In a letter from my father just a few months before I met Jim, he mentioned that my mother had not been able to reconcile the fact that I had married someone beneath me, that is, someone "stupid and poor." Of course, that wasn't true, but then, my life had not followed my mother's expectations, presuming that I would marry well, perhaps a doctor or a lawyer. In his letter, my father expressed relief that no one had inquired about me, otherwise my mother would, no doubt, blame him for her "unbearable suffering." If she had any inkling of Jim's medical history, my mother would quickly distance herself further and my father would be blamed again.

I often wondered if I was a disappointment to my mother. It's not as if I didn't try to earn her love. I got good grades at school, played the violin in the elementary school orchestra and dutifully practiced the piano. Perhaps I wasn't quite the protégé that my mother hoped for, since she never came to any of the recitals when I performed at the Royal Conservatory of Music. After all, I was 11, and old enough to go on my own. Besides, she had heard me play Beethoven's *Für Elise* countless times. Still, my mother made sure I was wearing my best dress, my shoes properly polished, my hair neatly braided and there were two streetcar tickets in my little purse.

All the other children were sitting with their parents. I just explained to my teacher that my father was working out of town and my mother was too busy to come, with newborn twins and a little sister at home. It was the same story when I ended up in the ER at Sick Kids

Hospital with a broken wrist after falling while ice skating with friends after school.

Now, I was alone again and only had myself to blame.

Perhaps I should have bailed out weeks ago. In fact, I should never have let Jim move in, not when he was worried about the Mafia following him. And to think, I just laughed. Was I as crazy as he was? Still, the first few weeks were wonderful. I had never met someone who was so devoted to me and interested in my dreams. He pushed all the right buttons, and I was flying high as well. How could I have possibly known that Jim had a history of severe mental illness? And that his descent into madness began soon after we met?

The following morning, I dragged myself out of bed and called in sick, taking the rest of the week off to recover. I cleaned up my apartment and stashed Jim's personal belongings into the closet. I covered up my bruises with some make-up and went to the hospital.

The psychiatric wing was very demoralizing with patients shuffling back and forth along the hallways. A nurse took me to the isolation room where Jim had been placed when he became aggressive toward some of the other patients. There was a small window in the locked door and I could see Jim sleeping on a bare cot in the corner. He had lost weight during his manic month, and looked so small, helpless and harmless, in an oversized pair of hospital PJs.

Jim had been given an injection, no doubt, Haldol (haloperidol), to calm him down. Despite its harmful side effects, the powerful neuroleptic, discovered by Paul Janssen in 1958, was indispensable in psychiatric emergencies. The nurse kindly suggested that I come back the next day: "Hopefully, he won't be as heavily sedated then."

I left the hospital in a daze and drove to the airport to pick up Jim's father. A huge weight lifted off my shoulders when he gave me an awkward hug. Although we barely knew each other, I felt so very comfortable in his presence. After checking him into the hotel, we went to a small neighbourhood bistro for dinner. There was so much to talk about. But first, we ordered a good bottle of wine. It would be a long evening.

Unconditional love

I learned that Jim had been hospitalized several times, with his father always on hand to make sure that he had access to the very best medical care, both in the United States and Canada. Although his parents failed to understand how a mental illness could create such havoc in their lives, they never gave up on Jim.

In mid-December 1965, Jim's father drove to Hanover, New Hampshire, to pick him up from Mary Hitchcock Memorial Hospital. Jim had been attending Canaan College in a nearby town working toward a Bachelor of Arts degree, when he became severely depressed. In a letter to his father, Jim wrote about his inability to find purpose in life and the difficulties he was having as far as meeting his course requirements. His father wrote back providing the following assurances:

When you get home for the holidays, we can have a full discussion of the problem and in the meantime get the thoughts of going completely insane out of your mind... You mention that at this point in life you have not really established a purpose in being alive... Just how many people your age could say they have established a purpose? For that matter, how many middle-aged people could say that?

I think you underrate yourself a great deal Jim and if you could only have more faith in your ability. I think you would be surprised with the results you could obtain... Just remember that we all want to help you. Just let us know your problems and I am sure we can lick them together.

The timing of Jim's hospitalization, so far away from home, could not have been worse. His mother had just been released after a 46-day stay at Toronto General Hospital and was still recovering from a severe depressive episode. When she was recuperating from a hysterectomy in early October, the nursing staff became alarmed when they discovered her talking non-stop on the phone, placing bets with a bookie on horse races. Although her uncle Col. H.R. Marshall was president of the Ontario Jockey Club for many years and his horse Blue Light had won the prestigious Queen's Plate in 1961, she had never shown any interest in horses, or gambling, for that matter.

Her bizarre behaviour took everyone by surprise since she was a quiet, rather reserved woman who was always careful with her money.

Jim's mother was transferred to the psychiatric ward and heavily sedated with private nurses hired to keep an eye on her, 24 hours a day. It is not uncommon for sudden hormonal changes to trigger severe mood swings for women, especially if there is an inherited predisposition for mental illness. Back then, there was no knowledge of the unique genetic risk factors and shared clinical characteristics of manic-depressive illness. It was no secret that her father Noel Clifford Marshall, a wealthy businessman, was an alcoholic. There was never any shame associated with his excessive alcohol consumption; not like there would be with a family member living with a mental illness. That message was obvious in the following note to Jim from his father following his mother's ECT (electroconvulsive therapy) treatments.

He (the doctor) told me that she would not remember anything that happened prior to the treatments and said that it would be better if we did not discuss it in the future. I think she realizes that she has been sick but certainly does not realize how serious it was.

There was no question that Jim's condition was just as serious since he was subsequently hospitalized at Toronto Psychiatric Hospital for another six weeks. According to a medical report, Jim was suffering from "elective mutism," as well as severe anxiety and depression. His prognosis was poor, and a recommendation was made for psychotherapy. Jim's efforts to get his life back on track were unsuccessful. He saw a psychiatrist on a weekly basis for almost two months, without any marked improvement in his overall disposition. He enrolled for some non-credit courses at the University of Toronto, but they didn't provide any direction as far as potential career opportunities.

That summer, Jim managed to get a job at the historic Algonquin Resort, St. Andrews-by-the-Sea, in New Brunswick. A former junior member of the Toronto Golf Club, he was assigned to assist in the pro shop for its golf course, famous for its spectacular views of the

Atlantic Ocean. Admittedly, the position was a relatively easy one, for someone with an upbeat disposition, and a sound knowledge of the sport. Jim, however, was already depressed when he arrived at the resort. A minor accident with his Volvo further deepened his sense of despair. Although he was not injured, and there was very little damage to the car, Jim became anxious and fearful. When he started to experience auditory and visual hallucinations, Jim locked himself into his motel room and called his father, asking him to come to St. Andrews and drive him home.

Jim spent the next four weeks at Homewood Sanatorium, at the time, a private psychiatric facility north of Toronto. The diagnosis when he was admitted, according to the medical record, was catatonic schizophrenia, a rare disorder, describing his inability to respond events around him. Jim's memories of his stay are vague, but he remembers that the food was much better than typical hospital fare and there were always cloth napkins on the table for every meal. After he was discharged, Jim took the time to write to Dr. Arthur, thanking him and referencing the eight ECT treatments he had received while under his care:

Just a short note to thank you for your assistance beyond the call of duty... My stay was highly beneficial to my health and my future plans... I was not aware of how sick I was, until I was told what a remarkable change there was in my attitude towards other people after I had the treatments. I am also pleased with my quick recovery and the wonderful way I feel and look now.

Jim's father had already endured so much heartache over his son's illness and now, he was faced with the cruel reality of another relapse with him so far from home. Nevertheless, for the first time, Jim had a proper diagnosis of a mental illness that had stymied many in the medical profession for years. I tried to be optimistic, sharing the information about the promising new drug lithium, an important breakthrough in the treatment of mood disorders.

And yet, I remained cautious, desperately missing the kind, gentle person that I fell in love with, but still fearful that Jim might turn on me again, driven by an unknown force beyond my understanding.

Payne Whitney Psychiatric Clinic

The following morning, we went to visit Jim. He had been transferred to a room and was awake, but still quite groggy from the medication. At any rate, Jim seemed very pleased that we had come to see him. He had some recollection of the events prior to his hospitalization, and was able to provide us with clues, as far as retrieving his belongings. We found his car at Lincoln Center and returned it to the rental agency. We also tracked down Skull's Angels, the cab company based in Queen's, and managed to retrieve the box of personal papers he had left in the car. I called the Cathedral hoping to locate his jacket, shoes and his prized Mont Blanc fountain pen, but they were nowhere to be found.

A few days later, Jim was transferred to the small private 100-bed facility with a country club atmosphere and a VIP suite for celebrities. Journalist Jane Pauley, host of *Sunday Morning* on CBS television, wrote about her stay in her biography, *Skywriting, a Life Out of the Blue*, when she was suffering from wild mood swings.

Jim's private room was sparsely furnished, looking more like a room in a college dorm than a typical hospital ward. The rules were strict; no visitors for the first two weeks, and then, it was only on Wednesday afternoons and weekends. The focus was on patient care and Jim has always believed that the move to Payne Whitney saved his life.

At the time, there was very little information about manic-depressive illness considering that the first documented diagnosis of the mental disorder appeared in an 1851 article, when a French psychiatrist Jean-Pierre Falret described the shifts in mood he observed in people, alternating between manic excitement and severe depression, as *la folie circularie*, which translates as "a circular madness."

I also learned that Jim was in good company, as far as his diagnosis was concerned. Many of our most talented writers, artists, composers and statesmen, who have enriched our lives, also suffered from extremes of elation and despair. In spite of this, I continued to have doubts about a future with Jim.

I would learn soon enough that the lack of financial and personal responsibility were symptoms of the illness. I had no idea how I was going to deal with such a quandary, when it was highly unlikely that Jim could change his habits, even if he promised to do so. I was completely in the dark about Jim's finances. I had just assumed that he could afford the extravagant lifestyle that we were enjoying. Jim never asked me to contribute, when we dined out at neighbourhood restaurants, and I never offered. Besides, he was essentially living rent-free in my apartment. Although we shared many common traits, we may as well have lived on different planets, when it came to handling our personal finances. I was careful with each pay cheque, focusing on paying bills and putting some savings aside, so I could afford the occasional purchase from Bloomingdale's and other high-end department stores. Jim, on the other hand, never expressed any concerns about the price of a bottle of wine or a ticket for a Broadway musical.

Although I visited Jim often during his five-week stay at Payne Whitney, I kept a very tight grip on my emotions. Jim was remorseful of his treatment of me in the days prior to his hospitalization and hopeful that we could rekindle the love we shared, when he was well enough to come home. Always resourceful, Jim managed to find a typewriter and wrote extensively about the events of the past month.

It is very hard at times to deal with reality in an unreal atmosphere, spending one's day in a protected hospital is hardly a real situation...the past few weeks are a bit confusing. I do recall most of the events that led up to it but there are a few gaps still... I had an agenda. Lembi was very distressed when she learned I had handed in my resignation. I was getting more and more agitated by her comments. I had to be in control. Why was she giving me such a hard time? We got into an argument and I slapped her across the face to shut her up.

One thing for sure what I did at St Patrick's I would never again attempt to do, nor would I dare think of treating Lembi in the manner which I did on that day... It is of little consequence at this time whether or not I am supposed to represent God or not. I have too many real-life situations to deal with concerning myself, Lembi and our future together.

Lembi is it for the rest of my life. I want to marry her and have children and grandchildren. I do see a life ahead full of happiness… the future is ours if we want it. If we don't that too is our decision. So let it be.

Although Jim was responding well to the lithium trials, I still had grave concerns about Jim's state of mind, especially after reading about the specific details that led to his hospitalization:

The truth of the matter is I had some very good reasons for the events at St. Patrick's. Initially when I entered the Cathedral, I was looking for Cardinal Cooke. I wanted to have a talk with him regarding unification of churches under the title of catholic (not R.C.) --- meaning universal. After listening to a Mass, I said confession… I was told to seek out what I was looking for.

After his confession with a priest, Jim found his way to the Chancel Organ located beside the high alter on the main level of the Cathedral. He sat down on the bench, took off his jacket, shoes and socks and laid them down on the floor.

I was almost tempted to try and play it - I should have - then I would have been kicked out of the Cathedral - not letting the door open to future events… I decided to continue my quest. People were very helpful in pointing directions out to me. So I continued over to the south side of the church to a door which led upward to a set of stairs which I climbed. On the third level, I got hold of a fire extinguisher and hurled it over on the alter, activated, as a blessing.

Six miles of scaffolding had been erected inside the Cathedral on September 26, 1972, to brace the ceiling from possible harmful effects of blasting of a construction site across the street. According to an article in the *Daily News*, dated April 19, 1973, "…more than 100 cleaners, painters and plasterers had been scurrying up the 100-foot-high platforms in a nine-month long 'sprucing up' of the landmark's 95-year-old history."

I climbed stair after stair until I banged my way through a couple of boards and found myself on the scaffolding. What a freak-out. At this point I went through a number of things which would hopefully lead me to meeting the Cardinal. I shorted fuse boxes (high voltage). It was really fascinating - then I continued on my way - further upward.

I eventually found my way to the top - the roof - which I climbed up on - and walked over several areas. At this point I was waiting for a helicopter to take me to God. There were two workmen who started to shout at me. They led me back down through the Cathedral to an exit on the south side where two of New York's finest were waiting for me.

Fortunately for Jim, the police took him to Metropolitan Hospital, with one of the largest mental health facilities in the city. Things could have been much worse, if he had been taken to the local police precinct on a mischief charge.

Credit card crisis

When Jim was discharged from Payne Whitney, he went back to Toronto to stay with his parents for the time being. Truth be told, I needed more time to sort out my own future. Prior to meeting me, Jim had never experienced a manic episode accompanied by a psychotic break with reality. Nor was there any previous evidence of violent behaviour. Now, we were dealing with the unknown. I continued to have doubts about a future relationship with someone who had already been hospitalized on numerous occasions for severe disturbances in mood. Would I be able to arrange psychiatric care for him, if there was another crisis?

Just as disturbing, was Jim's history of indiscriminate spending sprees relying on credit cards to pay for a lifestyle that he could ill afford. Would Jim continue his extravagant ways now that he no longer had a job? My own financial position was very modest with no room for major unexpected expenses. Jim's father reimbursed me for the cost having the locks changed, as well as my excessive phone bill, that included late-night, long-distance calls by Jim to a family friend living in Hawaii.

Neither of us were aware that Jim was heavily in debt to five New York banks. During dinner one night when he was still in New York, Jim's father, a former bank manager, shared his frustrations of how he had tried for years to advise his son about finances. I was stunned to discover that Jim had essentially squandered a sizable inheritance

63

from his grandmother when he was 21 years old and still living at home. Jim bought a Lotus Elan +2, a pricey British sports car, but he realized soon enough, that he couldn't afford the maintenance for an engine that needed to be tuned with the aid of a stethoscope. When his real estate investment in four townhouses (with first and second mortgages) failed to generate the income needed to cover expenses, his father refused to bail him out. Instead, he managed to negotiate a settlement with the bank and his mother wrote the cheque to pay off the debt.

Jim had already told me about the loss of the townhouses; he was very bitter about his parents' reluctance to provide the necessary funds to protect his investments. "They could have taken the money out of my future inheritance," he complained. "Think of what the townhouses would be worth today." I didn't say anything, but I thought that Jim was being unreasonable. First, he refused to accept responsibility for poor judgment and secondly, he was transferring the blame for his failure to his parents, which I found to be troublesome. I realized that I had no choice but to maintain my financial independence. Unknown to me at the time, the decision was a fortuitous one, since one of the most common symptoms of bipolar disorder is compulsive and irresponsible spending.

However, there were more urgent questions than dealing with financial matters. What about the volatile shifts in mood? Would I be putting myself in danger again, if Jim became irritable, angry and paranoid? How would the stigma of mental illness impact our lives and our children's lives? What about future employment? Jim had resigned from his job at "Ma Bell" during a manic episode; and so, it was extremely doubtful that he would receive a decent reference from his former employer, the New York Telephone Company. How would we support ourselves in the interim?

As it was, I had yet to let my parents or sisters know that Jim had been hospitalized. I certainly didn't expect them to understand my predicament. My friends were skeptical as well. No one was rallying around me providing any support, not the way people comfort a friend who's loved one was living with a serious cancer diagnosis.

Back then, I wasn't aware of any support groups for people living with mental illness or their family members, not like Alcoholics Anonymous and Al-Anon, with many of its members, no doubt, self-medicating because of a genetic predisposition of bipolar disorder for abusing alcohol.

Picking up the pieces

As spring approached, I was invited by Jim's father to join them for a week at Myrtle Beach in South Carolina. They would drive down from Toronto and I could fly from New York to meet them. Perhaps some time together without any distractions would give us a chance to see if we were really destined to spend the rest of our lives together. I was anxious, but then, who wouldn't be?

There was Jim, smiling as I walked into the airport and into his arms. He held me for a long time in a tender embrace and all the wonderful feelings I had felt for Jim during the early days of our relationship flooded back in that moment. We were so happy back then, deliriously happy, as we planned our future together. I had to be honest with my emotions. I was still very much in love with Jim.

We spent much of the time walking along the beach, holding hands, and rediscovering each other. We decided that we really did have a great deal in common and so, there was every reason to be optimistic. The hardships we had experienced and overcome only strengthened our resolve to commit to each other. I was also assured by the love Jim's father had for his son, and comforted by the realization that I, too, could lean on him for support in the weeks and months ahead. Also, the knowledge that the manic episode Jim experienced could now be prevented with medication, provided us with the confidence and a sense of security to trust the love Jim and I had for each other.

Lithium is truly a wonder drug, a major chemical breakthrough, in the treatment of manic-depressive illness. Approved in 1970 by the Food and Drug Administration in United States, the naturally occurring simple salt, lithium carbonate, found in mineral water and rock formations, acts as a mood stabilizer. It is available as a capsule and costs pennies per dose. Lithium continues to be the gold standard for the treatment of the abnormal brain functioning that cause extreme mood swings. Researchers believe that lithium helps strengthen nerve cell connections in the brain involved in regulating mood, thinking and behaviour to maintain the equilibrium between highs and lows.

We returned to New York together and began planning our move to Nova Scotia. I still owned a small, winterized cottage on Peggy's Cove Road, 30 kilometres outside of Halifax that my ex-husband and I had purchased in 1970. It was an idyllic spot on the waterfront with four acres of land, mostly wooded and very private.

Although there was no question that Jim was very ill when he wrote his resignation letter to his previous employer, he was fearful that the stigma would have been too great for him to return to the office as an ex-psychiatric patient. If Jim was an alcoholic requiring a month's stay at a rehab clinic, he would have been welcomed back provided additional assistance if needed under the company's Employee Assistance Program. If he required considerable rehab after a motor vehicle accident, the same assistance was available. People diagnosed with a serious mental illness were treated differently.

Jim and I were married in New York on December 1, 1973, at the Church of the Holy Trinity, the Episcopal congregation in our neighbourhood. Jim's parents flew down for the wedding and our friends held a reception for us in their home. We toasted our future with a bottle of Moët & Chandon Champagne from France, an extravagance, to be sure, but it was a special day and Jim had to have the very best.

Our only gifts to each other were the 18K gold engraved wedding bands from Tiffany & Company. For better, for worse, for richer, for poorer, in sickness, and in health, we were now ready to embrace the new "normal" of our lives.

Chapter Three - The New Normal

St. Margarets Bay, Nova Scotia

A brand-new chapter in our relationship was about to begin with the roller coaster on standby, ready to rev up again when we least expected it. Once again, there were no alarm bells warning me that my world would come crashing down, leaving me frightened and facing an uncertain future.

Starting all over again was tough. Nevertheless, Jim was very resourceful and managed to get through job interviews without disclosing a history of mental illness that had interrupted his educational and career prospects all too often. He found a temporary position that summer with the Canadian government as an information officer, promoting a program designed to assist farmers throughout the Maritime Provinces. Then, Jim found a permanent position as an education and information officer with the Nova Scotia Credit Union League, a not-for-profit organization that provided administrative support for credit unions across the province. The following year, Jim was promoted to the position of director of communications for the League.

Our lives were back on track. We could not have been happier although our rural lifestyle was very low key after all the excitement of New York. At the same time, we missed the city and the Sunday morning ritual of reading *The New York Times*. I framed our favourite *New Yorker* magazine covers and hung them in our bathroom. We watched *Kojak* just to see the familiar street scenes on the popular TV cop show.

Jonathan was born soon after we moved to St. Margarets Bay and Larissa arrived two years later. I had always wanted children and they brought immeasurable joy to our lives. I loved being a mom. I was determined that my children would always know that they were special. On the other hand, I don't remember my own mother feeling anything more than a sense of duty when caring for her own five daughters. Nor did she express any joy with the birth of her grandchildren. I was deeply disappointed when there were no congratulatory cards, no flowers, no gifts, no nothing, not on their first birthdays nor at Christmas. I am not sure if I was still being punished for a failed first marriage and I didn't ask. I knew that my mother never approved of Jim, especially when she found out about his hospitalization, when we still lived in New York. It seems that the stigma of mental illness in the family must have been even more terrifying for her than the stigma of a daughter's divorce.

Perhaps, I shouldn't be so hard on my own mother. When I was born in Okelbo, a small town just outside of Gavle, Sweden, where we lived, my parents weren't married. They were refugees meeting in a neutral country, while the war still raged across Europe. Estonia was occupied first by the Russians, then the Germans, when my father managed to escape as a stowaway on a freighter headed across the Baltic Sea to Finland. My mother escaped later in a small boat with two brothers and two sisters when the Russians bombed Tallinn and rolled across the border with their tanks. Both suffered from symptoms of post-traumatic stress disorder (PTSD), but they never made the correlation that their suffering might be similar to some of Jim's frightening hallucinations when he was ill.

By the time we were settled in Nova Scotia, Jim had fully recovered. He was seen on a regular basis by a psychiatrist in Halifax and continued to take lithium to prevent future psychotic episodes. As far as I knew, Jim was always compliant taking his medication, and there was no reason to be concerned. Just the same, I was hyper-vigilant, watching for any signs or symptoms that might suggest that all was not well. By now, there was more literature on manic-depressive illness. I read everything I could about this fascinating and yet, destructive medical condition of the human brain that threatened to push the lives of highly productive, creative and talented people off the rails. How that happens remains a mystery to this day.

When his boss, the manager of the League passed away suddenly in March 1978 from a heart attack, Jim had difficulty adjusting to the loss. Fortunately, his low mood was short-lived, and I breathed a sigh of relief. Now that Jim was feeling better, I was more concerned about my own well-being, feeling tired much of the time and seeing a specialist because of a suspected case of endometriosis. The children had also been sick with colds that winter, further draining my limited physical resources.

Suddenly, it was spring, and our moods reflected the joyous renewal of my favourite time of year. Our Canadian winters were harsher and lasted longer than what we experienced in New York, but soon the days were sunny and warm. The snow, still deep in our woods, had almost disappeared. It wouldn't be long before the daffodils would fight their way through the frozen ground to the surface, symbols of the joy and happiness we felt so deeply.

On Easter Sunday, we attended the service at All Saints Cathedral in Halifax which had an excellent pipe organ. Jim wasn't particularly religious, but he enthusiastically joined the congregation during the singing of the hymns with a rich and melodic voice that was note perfect despite his inability to read music.

The following weekend, we were back at the Cathedral for the Sunday service. During the singing of the contemporary hymn, *Lord of the Dance* by Sydney Carter, Jim quickly became very animated, practically dancing to the lively music as the children joined in, standing up on the pew and clapping their hands.

I did not realize it at the time, that the hymn's first-person portrayal of the life and mission of Jesus Christ posed serious harm for someone like Jim who could become preoccupied with God during periods of unpredictable mood swings. The lyrics were the trigger that would send him into another realm that was impossible for ordinary mortals to comprehend.

We had planned to spend a quiet evening at home. Just after 4:00 pm, however, Jim decided to go to the office and finish a proposal for his boss regarding an upcoming regional conference. He often put in extra time on weekends, so there was no reason for me to worry. I was proud of Jim, admiring his sense of commitment to the job. I would feed the children and put them to bed, and serve dinner when Jim came home later in the evening.

It never occurred to me that something was wrong until Jim left, with his briefcase, still dressed casually, wearing a pair of jeans and a sports shirt. Jim had always been a very conservative dresser, so I was surprised that he hadn't changed, or at the very least, put on a decent pair of chinos, before showing up at the office. There was that niggling feeling that something was not quite right.

I decided to act on my instincts and started to look for his medication. When I couldn't find his container of lithium in his drawer, or in the medicine cabinet in the bathroom, I panicked. I didn't know what to do and I didn't have anyone to turn to for advice. None of our friends knew of Jim's psychiatric history. We were always fearful of the stigma associated with mental illness, that we would be ostracized, and our children would be without friends.

Although it was Sunday evening, I managed to get hold of Jim's psychiatrist who confirmed my fears as I tried to recall the events of the previous week, and the ever so subtle symptoms of mania that morning at church. Dr. Rosenberg mentioned that he had not seen Jim in several months and suspected that he might need to be hospitalized. Unfortunately, medical intervention would be the last thing on someone's mind when he or she was feeling better than they have been in weeks, even months. Didn't Jim just say sometime last week that he was feeling "on top of the world?"

I tried to reach Jim at the office but there was no answer. Considering the state I was in, I was not about to call his parents. Not yet, anyway. I was not only anxious but also afraid. In fact, I was terrified. By then, I was frantic with worry and kept fighting back my tears. I didn't want to cry in front of the children who needed to be fed their dinner and put to bed. We recently celebrated Jonathan's fourth birthday and Larissa was only 18 months old. Jim was a very gentle person who loved his children dearly, and would never intend to hurt them. Unfortunately, I knew better. I was aware how he could become hostile, paranoid, and possibly violent, if he was delusional while on a mission responding to a higher authority.

Was it my fault?

I was angry at myself for not recognizing the changes in mood, however insignificant they may have been at the time. Why didn't I see through his overly optimistic outlook and realize that some of it was just too good to be true? How could I be fooled by my own husband? Shouldn't I have known better? Shouldn't he have known better when his medication ran out and seen his psychiatrist right away? Surely, he had some responsibility as far as keeping his appointments, or was it my responsibility as well?

My stress level was extreme. Our house was set back from the highway with dense woods in between. It would be impossible to escape with two toddlers, if Jim came home in a psychotic state. I called Debbie, a friend who lived nearby and asked her to come over and help with the children. While waiting for her, I raced around the house, hiding everything that might be sharp, all our knives, my sewing scissors, even my knitting needles.

While Debbie fed Jonathan and Larissa, I tried to think through my next steps. My priority was keeping the children safe and I asked Debbie to take them for the night. As good friends often do, she tried to reassure me that everything would be fine and suggested that I might be exaggerating my fears. After all, she knew Jim better than most of our friends. He had taught Debbie to drive whenever her husband, a fisheries officer, was away at sea. Strange as it may seem, he objected to her having a driver's licence. Debbie certainly knew exactly how patient Jim could be, as she struggled to learn to drive a car with standard transmission without stripping the gears.

I dressed the children and packed their essentials, a few toys, Jonathan's Snoopy and Larissa's precious Lolly Dolly. We walked over to Debbie's house, and I hugged them for a long time. I just didn't know how soon I would see them again. I also had to implore Debbie not to let Jim into the house, if he came looking for me or the children. How could I explain to her that I was afraid that he might kidnap, or worse, harm them?

Alone at home and waiting to hear from Jim became unbearable. I tried calling his office again, hoping that all my fears were unfounded. When there was no response, I called one of his closest friends, someone Jim had known when they were both still living in Toronto. Barry lived nearby with his wife Donna, and without any hesitation, he agreed to come right over. I tried to explain why I was so worried as I recounted his manic episode in New York five years earlier, when Jim escaped near death while climbing the scaffolding at St. Patrick's Cathedral all the way up to the roof. I knew that Jim, with an exaggerated sense of well-being and under the pressure of an extraordinary imagination was capable of anything, even defying the laws of gravity.

Like everyone else in our circle of friends, Barry was unaware of my husband's history of mental illness. That's hardly surprising considering how Jim's parents also managed to guard his secret from family and friends. The stigma alone could threaten his aspirations for a rewarding career.

Just after 11:00 pm, the phone rang. I suspected right away that it might be Jim. For the first time that evening, I tried to be calm. I didn't want Jim to think that I suspected anything to be amiss. Most of all, I didn't want him to feel threatened in any way. As it turned out, the phone call was a charade. When I started to ask questions, Jim assured me that there was nothing to worry about and that he would be home soon. "Trust me," he said, ending the call abruptly and hanging up. The last time, Jim said, "Trust me," he was already certifiably mentally ill. I still didn't know where he was since I half expected him to be on his way home.

"Please God," I prayed, "let Jim be OK." There had been no indication of the unusual behaviour or volatile mood swings which had been the case when we lived in New York. Sure, Jim was sad when his former boss died unexpectedly. That seemed to be, at least to me, a normal response. But now, I knew better. The pendulum had swung in the opposite direction and Jim was headed for another psychotic break. I spent the night at Barry's house.

The following morning, I went back home. When Jim's car was still missing from the garage, I called the RCMP and filed a missing person's report with Sergeant Kelly. I dreaded having to be honest about Jim's history of mental illness but there was no choice, since he could pose a danger to himself and others if he was psychotic. I also called Dave, one of Jim's friends at work, but he hadn't heard from him either. An hour later, Dave called back to advise me that Jim had just been in touch with the office, saying that he was home sick with the flu.

So where was he?

A perfect life

Looking back, the past few weeks had been almost perfect. Jim was more relaxed than he had been in long time, despite the pressures at work and his relentless drive to be successful. Jim had almost finished putting together the corporate annual report for the League's 50th anniversary with gold leaf on the cover, featuring historical photos as well as bios of some of the early board members. He was also responsible for the monthly newsletter and arranging for radio and television advertising. Jim had incredible insight, almost a sixth sense, as far as understanding the nuances of the corporate culture and how best to promote the growth of member credit unions. His exceptional writing skills, along with seemingly endless reserves of energy, were invaluable assets for someone in his position, in a very competitive field.

Jim was also more attentive to my needs. On the previous Saturday morning, Jim was up early, and had coffee ready before I got up. He had made breakfast for the children and expressed some concern about not spending enough time with them. I was happy when he decided to take Jonathan to the movies that afternoon, since it would be a rare treat for both.

On his way home, Jim had picked up a special bottle of wine, and we dined alone after the children were put to bed. It was almost like falling in love all over again, the two of us, sipping our wine and holding hands across the table. The past was the past. We rarely talked about the turmoil in our lives created by circumstances beyond our control. We were grateful for the advances in medicine that gave Jim a new lease on life and a promising future for our family.

I often told my friends that I was one of the luckiest people in the world. I had a husband who adored me, and we had two exceptional children. Jim was also a genius in the kitchen, creating gourmet meals from basic ingredients stocked in our cupboards. A box of Kraft Dinner was transformed into a culinary delight for Jonathan and Larissa. So, it came as no surprise when Jim won *Chatelaine* magazine's "Entertaining Spectacular" category in an annual cooking contest for his eggplant parmigiana recipe in January 1976. The $100 prize went toward an original Alexander Calder lithograph that has always hung on the wall of our dining room.

As I looked back at the last few weeks searching for clues of an imminent psychotic relapse, there were no red flags or alarm bells. Despite the heavy odds stacked up against him from an early age, Jim managed to maintain a very positive perspective on life. Sure, there were days when his mood was low, particularly when another rejection letter arrived in the mail. Somehow, we managed to scrape by on my meagre savings and much-appreciated financial support from Jim's parents, Once Jim's position at the League was secure, we bought a new Volvo station wagon, which we named "Albert," an addition to "Bertha," a special edition yellow VW Super Beetle, bought when we were still living in New York.

Jim had also encouraged me to consider a career as a writer, so that I could stay home with the children. Although I was an avid reader, I had never dared to dream of becoming an author, considering the dismal grades in my English composition classes. I was skeptical at first, but Jim was convinced that I could be successful, and as always, he was right.

We had a few new regional magazines, so I was fortunate to have a local market for my stories and photographs. I borrowed books on journalism from the library in Halifax and studied them, and made notes, as if I was tackling a complicated experiment in the chemistry lab at university. Jim proved to be a tough critic and I owe him a great deal of gratitude for not giving up on me while the trash can beside the typewriter on the dining room table kept filling up with endless rewrites.

My early articles appeared in several magazines, including *Sea Frontiers*, published by the International Oceanographic Foundation, in Florida. I also had a contract sourcing photographs and illustrations for the 18-volume series, *Canada's Illustrated Heritage* with Pierre Berton at its helm. I even managed to get a few gigs as a reporter for a CBC radio morning show, specializing in news items related to discoveries in science and medicine.

Now my own story was unfolding.

Lost Hills, California

The phone call I feared most came late Monday evening.

It was Jim.

At first, I was happy to hear his voice since he sounded fine. That was before I learned that he was calling from the other side of the continent, almost 5,000 kilometres away, and in urgent need of medical care. Still, I was struck by his relatively calm demeanour as if he was just out of town on a business trip. Jim explained that he had checked into the Howard Johnson's Motel on the outskirts of Los Angeles and was waiting for me and the children to join him; he had already put in a request for a crib for Larissa. Jim gave me the address for the motel and asked me to come as soon as possible.

I was afraid to say much, worried that Jim might become suspicious and take off again. I tried to ask him what he was doing in Los Angeles, but he promised to explain everything as soon as I arrived. Apparently, Jim never went to the office on Sunday afternoon and drove straight to the airport. He had been smart enough to pack his $400 Halston Ultrasuede blazer into his briefcase and probably looked reasonably respectable when purchasing his airline tickets. Nor did anyone question the fact that he had no luggage to check.

First, Jim boarded a flight for Montreal, then Toronto, spending the night at the Howard Johnson's Airport Hotel. The following morning, he flew to Los Angeles. While en route to the West Coast, he was already focusing on his next mission in life which he described in a letter, hoping to mail it to me when he arrived at his destination.

Trust that you saw Oral Roberts (televangelist) last night – knockout performance. What a changed man – really got the message across. By the time this reaches you, I trust that you will have a better understanding of my mission in life – I knew I couldn't be wrong! Sure, it is a dream – by God enjoy it!

Although Jim was flying high, literally, and figuratively, he still had the mental capacity to book his travel and behave, at least outwardly, in an acceptable, "normal" manner. Jim managed to enter the United States without raising any suspicions among both immigration and customs officers, considering he was travelling with an empty briefcase and an expired passport.

When Jim arrived in Los Angeles, he rented a car and drove straight to the motel. As he indicated in his letter, Jim was on a mission. He believed that as an envoy of God, he would be collecting a special Oscar at the Academy Awards ceremony that evening for his humanitarian deeds. When Jim was unable to contact the right person to confirm his invitation, Jim opened the mini bar, poured himself a double Scotch and called home.

I immediately got in touch with Sergeant Kelly at the RCMP, who notified the Los Angeles police, asking them to take Jim to the nearest hospital for a psychiatric evaluation. Not surprisingly, Jim refused to open the door when the police arrived. The fact that he was in mental distress did not give the police the legal authority to enter his room without a warrant, as long as Jim had not committed a crime. Instead, he grabbed his briefcase, unlocked the patio door and fled the motel in his rental car. Jim decided to drive home and headed out of town. As he later explained, "It seemed the logical thing to do under the circumstances."

When I learned that Jim had managed to evade the police, my heart sank. Just the same, the knowledge that Jim was still alive, calmed me enough to be able to sleep that night. With Jim so far away, it was also safe to bring Jonathan and Larissa back home in the morning. But I was still anxious, pacing around the house. I was also in touch with Jim's parents, keeping them posted with each new development. I could tell from our telephone calls that they were stressed out as well.

Dave called me later that morning, to let me know that Jim had made a collect call to the office and left a phone number for us to get in touch with him, along with the name of his lawyer in Halifax. I was now confronted with the anxiety-ridden task of explaining to Jim's new boss that he was not home in bed with the flu. And I still had to track him down.

Nervously, I dialed the number Jim had left with his office. I was caught off guard when a disarmingly cheerful voice of a nurse answered my call:

"Psychiatric ward. May I help you?"

I immediately breathed a sigh of relief. Jim was safe. That's all that mattered at that moment.

I explained that I was Jim's wife and the nurse put me on hold while she went to find him.

At first, Jim was upbeat, telling me that, "The asparagus they served at lunch was just amazing." One would think he was staying at a five-star resort. It may as well have been a posh hotel, considering the daily rate the hospital was charging. Any sense of reassurance that Jim might be OK was short-lived, when his mood suddenly darkened, as he lashed out at me. Jim was furious about being hospitalized against his will. And it was my job to get him out. He demanded that I call our lawyer, "who knows everything," for the details regarding his discharge. When I started asking questions, Jim abruptly hung up on me.

I later discovered that Jim's prescription for lithium had run out during a recent business trip to Montreal. When Jim returned home from the conference, he was too busy to see his psychiatrist. Besides, he was feeling fine. While he was still a patient at Payne Whitney, Jim had been advised that he might consider weaning himself off the drug, if he remained stable for five years. The concern was harmful long-term side effects of lithium, including kidney damage. Regardless of the reason to discontinue the drug, such action would require careful supervision by a doctor.

If only I had known.

I was angry.

Once again, I was robbed of the person I had fallen in love with. In his place was an arrogant, self-righteous, unstable individual who didn't care about anybody but himself. I called the hospital back and asked to speak with someone in charge. That was the beginning of countless long-distance calls during Jim's six-day stay in the psychiatric ward. The social worker assured me that Jim was agreeable as far as taking his medication and could be released as soon as he was well enough to travel.

I learned that Jim had been brought to Kern Medical Center in Bakersfield by the California Highway Patrol (CHP) and the circumstances of his hospitalization were covered in the local press. One of the patients had given Jim a copy of the article. According to the headline, "Canadian leads CHP on long chase" in the April 4, 1978, edition of *The Bakersfield Californian*, the pursuit began in Los Angeles.

An officer had attempted to pull Jim over, when his red Toyota Corolla illegally crossed into the centre lane, as he was trying to pass another car. However, Jim had no intention of stopping. Instead, he floored the gas pedal, speeding and weaving in and out of the traffic without incident. Other patrol cars joined the chase as Jim sped along Interstate 5, heading north, for more than 200 kilometres.

They chased the car at speeds of 95-100 miles per hour before the driver pulled over to the shoulder of Twisselman Road. When he stopped, the driver rolled up the windows, locked the doors and refused to come out on command, officers said. The engine of the man's car was still running so officer Bob Cave slashed three tires with a knife.

Jim explained that he had turned on his signal to pull over to the side of a desolate stretch of road near the town of Lost Hills, as soon as he realized he was running low on fuel. When the police pointed their rifles at him and ordered him out of the car, Jim was afraid that he might be killed as a martyr in his failed mission for God. Eventually, he got out of the car, was thrown to the ground, handcuffed, and searched for weapons.

When it was clear that Jim was not a criminal, the sergeant in charge suspected that he might be high on angel dust, a common name for phencyclidine, a psychedelic drug popular in the 1970s. Jim recalls being offered the choice of going to the police station or being taken to the hospital.

The circumstances of the "arrest," in the middle of nowhere, as the sun was setting, could have also been drastically different. Having a choice was pivotal, giving Jim a second chance. Otherwise, he could have been charged with impaired driving, reckless driving, and evading the police, all criminal violations in the state of California. In that case, Jim could be permanently barred from travelling to the United States.

There were serious problems facing us as far as getting Jim back home since he was not capable of travelling on his own. Although his company's health insurance policy with Blue Cross along with our provincial medical plan paid his hospital bills, there was no financial assistance available to bring him home.

Fortunately, Jim's credit card insurance covered the towing cost to return the rental car back to Los Angeles, as well as replacing the slashed tires. Jim was a skilled driver and there was no other damage to the car.

Deliver us from evil

After a week in the hospital, when Jim was relatively stable on his medications, his father travelled to California to bring him back to Nova Scotia. The psychiatric report was encouraging, and we hoped that he was well enough to recover at home.

We were wrong.

That night, Jim was restless and began pacing back and forth in our living room, pleading to God to save him from the evil forces inhabiting our home. It was impossible to turn off the delusional rantings of someone that neither of us recognized, a madman that had entered our lives uninvited and certainly not welcomed.

Jim finally went into the bedroom and closed the door. His father and I sat in the living room, keeping vigil all night. I had already blocked the door to the children's bedroom with heavy chairs and hoped for the best. I had also hidden the car keys to prevent Jim from taking off in the middle of the night.

The following morning, I called Jim's psychiatrist who advised me to bring him to the hospital as soon as possible. At first, he refused to go. As far as Jim was concerned, he was just having a bad reaction to the powerful psychotropic drugs given to him when he was hospitalized in California. Jim tried his best to assure us that he would be fine in a few days. No doubt, he was terrified about being locked up again. Jim also hated the side effects of Haldol, the tremors in his hands and the involuntary movement of his facial muscles. When we assured him that he should be home in a week, Jim finally agreed to go. Once again, we were so wrong.

Just when Jim seemed to be on the mend, he called me in the middle of the night, terrified that he was being poisoned by the staff. I had to come right away and rescue him. He had already called the local television station and left a message for the news anchor. It was a major setback for all of us.

While still delusional, Jim wrote several letters, though none were addressed to anyone. He rambled on about religion, life, love, happiness and family. His writing was very neat, and the sentence structures were sound. There was no indication that he was mentally ill except for his preoccupation with God when he confided that, "Jesus Christ himself was the devil. Hard to believe I bet. But take one moment to consider the world today."

Jim's father stayed with me while his son was hospitalized. He kept busy during the days working on our property and clearing a proper path to our beach. He also looked after Jonathan and Larissa when I visited Jim, who was still paranoid, suspicious of all visitors, including his own family. There simply are not enough words in the English language to describe the importance of his father's support that enabled me to get through such a difficult time with my sanity still intact.

Catastrophic job loss

We would learn soon enough that recovery from each psychotic episode becomes more complicated and takes longer. Together, Jim and I had climbed out of a big hole of despair that set in when he was hospitalized in New York in February 1973 without a job to go back to. This was no different.

Against the advice of his doctor, Jim went back to work within days of being released from the hospital on May 16. It was a fateful decision with disastrous consequences. If Jim had chosen to recuperate at home for another 30 days, his position might not have been in jeopardy.

But Jim was anxious to get back to work. There was the week-long regional conference in Antigonish with delegates from across the Maritime Provinces that he had helped organize. Jim felt that his presence was essential, though he had not fully recovered from his last psychotic episode.

In a letter to Jim's father dated May 23, I wrote: "The conference went quite well and there wasn't a soul there that didn't ask Jim how he was..." While it was obvious that Jim was well-liked and respected by his colleagues, all was not well. I noted that Jim was feeling low, concerned whether he could cope with the demands of his job: "I am sure this depression will pass, but it's making me a little nervous."

As it turned out, Jim had every reason to be anxious. Late in the afternoon on May 30, on Jim's second day back at the office after the conference, his boss, Jim McKinley walked into his office, handed him a letter and asked for his resignation.

Jim's recollection of that brief encounter was one of shock. "I wasn't given a choice." Mr. McKinley's letter only offered a modest severance package and raised serious questions regarding his motive:

I have been tempted in the past couple of months to let matters slide until the fall due to your recent illness. However, I don't feel that this course of action is in the best interest of the Nova Scotia Credit Union League or in the long-term for yourself.

After reading Mr. McKinley's letter, it was a wonder that Jim wasn't fired long ago. And yet, he had received annual salary increases since joining the company in October 1975, suggesting that he was a valued member of the staff. There was never any indication from management that his performance was unsatisfactory, not a single warning (written or otherwise) of incompetence or misconduct.

In any case, Jim's self-confidence was shattered.

The lowest blow was yet to come. A co-worker called the following day to advise Jim that the locks to the office had been changed. If he wished to pick up his personal belongings, someone would have to accompany him.

We needed to fight back though we suspected that the odds were against us. Jim contacted the Nova Scotia Human Rights Commission and provided a six-page response to Mr. McKinley's request for his resignation, addressing all the false allegations, and noting that there had never been any indication of dissatisfaction of his job performance.

It wasn't enough. Jim had to go.

In our experience, the stigma of mental illness was always more painful than the disease. Just as distressing was the fact that returning to work was crucial to Jim's well-being and recovery. He was blunt in his assessment of the loss of his PR position with the League: "They don't want a 'nut job' in an important communications slot."

Mr. McKinley may have been concerned about a court challenge when offering an increase in severance with the following caveat:

This extra compensation is intended to quicken the disposal of this matter and in no way indicates that we feel we may have been unjust in releasing Jim Buchanan as to timing, method or reasons.

We learned that people living with mental illnesses did not have the same rights as those living with physical disabilities. In Nova Scotia, the law had only recently recognized epilepsy as a physical condition eligible for disability benefits. But the provincial government continued to discriminate against people with a psychiatric diagnosis, notwithstanding the fact that manic-depressive illness is a medical condition caused by a similar chemical imbalance in the brain and treated with some of the same drugs as epilepsy. At the time, neither of us were prepared for a lengthy court battle.

There was nowhere else to turn.

Jim's self-esteem plummeted to a new low. The feelings of worthlessness and hopelessness were signs of the deep despair that had set in, and dominated our lives. For the first time, I was fearful that Jim might become suicidal.

Our birthdays came and went. Jonathan was disappointed when there was no cake on my birthday according to a brief notation in my journal on May 31. I made sure that there was cake and lots of candles for Jim's birthday on June 12. I had vowed, before our children were born, that I would shelter them as much as possible from the negative impacts of Jim's illness.

A beneficial and creative link

While there is a distinctive dark side to an illness that causes considerable damage to relationships and careers, there are also numerous beneficial aspects of this disease for some, creating a great deal of confusion when attempting to get a definitive diagnosis from a mental health practitioner. We are all familiar with the energy and drive, infectious enthusiasm, as well as artistic and creative elements, all packaged together, that has enabled many actors and musicians to achieve great success.

Patty Duke wrote about her personal experiences in a book titled, *A Brilliant Madness: Living with Manic-Depressive Illness,* co-authored with medical writer Gloria Hochman. Others include Mariah Carey, Carrie Fisher, Kurt Cobain, Demi Lovato, Jimi Hendrix and Vivien Leigh, to name a few.

That summer, I was fortunate to be involved with a major transformative commitment that kept me from being dragged down into a vortex of despair. As a fledgling member of the Canadian

Authors Association, I was on the committee hosting its annual national conference in Halifax at the end of June. The speakers and panelists of the five-day event were a who's who list of writers from across the country. I worked closely with my dear friend Joyce Barkhouse for almost a year, on many of the details in the planning process. Joyce was an author of a number of children's books, including, *Anna's Pet* which she co-wrote with her niece, Margaret Atwood. I was delighted, when invited by Joyce to join them for breakfast one morning at the Lord Nelson Hotel.

Our conference was a huge success and a good deal of credit goes to Jim. He had always been very intuitive, knowing exactly how to take advantage of local opportunities to benefit such an important gathering of literary talent in our province. Jim was able to guide me through a lot of the details in the early days of the planning process, as well as assist with press releases and other communication materials. He also encouraged me to trust my own instincts as far as coordinating social events and not to shy away from asking advertisers for generous contributions to pay for them.

While there were plenty of capable members of our association involved with the organization of the conference, I was able to fit right in, without any previous experience. When no one else wanted the job, I willingly volunteered to act as treasurer and pushed for a modest $5 increase in the registration fee, so we could include a lobster dinner for the attendees. After all, many of them had never been to Nova Scotia. When it was all over, we still had money left in our bank account, which we donated to the fledgling Writers' Federation of Nova Scotia for a scholarship fund.

The tide turns in our favour

Months passed before the gloom lifted, like the fog that penetrated St. Margarets Bay early on a summer morning, but receded once the sun came out in full force. By September, Jim was feeling well enough to resume an intensive job search. He was creative enough to fill in major gaps in his education and employment history. We remained confident that his skills would be recognized soon enough and that we could get our lives back on track.

Despite the many challenges that had threatened to sideline our marriage, we were still "crazy in love" with each other. Jim captured these sentiments in a hand-made card on a wedding anniversary:

As the years go by, I hope that we will learn to trust each other's feelings and hopefully meet each others' expectations of what life is really all about. I love you very much and I sincerely apologize for any selfish gaps in my personality.

Much love, Jim

The following spring, Jim was still unemployed and earnestly looking for a job, sending out dozens of resumés across the country. We were prepared to move if necessary. By now, I was a feature writer for *Halifax* magazine, but the pay was very modest, even when I was appointed its managing editor that summer. I had managed to find an excellent day care facility in the city for Jonathan and Larissa. Our financial position was extremely tight, but we managed to get by.

When Jim's 95-year-old grandfather passed away in June and left a small inheritance to Jim and the children, I thought that it might be a good time to have a discussion about our finances. Until then, I had been hesitant to bring up the subject since earlier attempts had threatened to create a rift in our relationship. But Jim had no interest in setting up a joint bank account, certainly not when he had significant cash reserves on hand. He continued to cover our major expenses while I looked after my personal needs, as well as those of the children. We remained poles apart when it came to managing our money.

I wasn't aware that Jim's father had asked him to hand over his credit cards when he lost his job with the New York Telephone in 1973. As a goodwill gesture, he would make monthly payments on Jim's debt until he found gainful employment. Although his father did not have the legal authority to cancel these accounts, he tried as he had so many times before, to instill a sense of financial responsibility in his wayward son. I probably should have paid more attention, when he copied me on the letter addressed to Jim, as we were packing up to move to Nova Scotia:

Lots of luck with your endeavours in Halifax. The going will be tough for the next year or two but you really have something to live for. It can't be any tougher than the past few years... I only ask you not to borrow but pay your way from day to day even if it means really skimping for a period of time... charge accounts are not the answer as you well know.

Back then, neither of us were aware that the insatiable need for credit cards to fuel extravagant spending sprees has always been one of the distressing hallmarks of bipolar disorder (as manic-depressive illness was renamed in 1980). During the next ten years, Jim's credit card collection continued to grow. Not that he needed all of them. We both had very good jobs and could afford the necessities of life, with plenty to spare. Regardless, Jim still managed to rack up quite a tab as I discovered, by chance, when the Xpresspost envelope from home landed on my hospital bed, as I was recovering from cancer surgery.

Chapter Four – Cancer Crisis

Grave consequences

Christmas has always been my favourite time of year. But the events leading up to the holidays in December 1990 would betray a sacred trust, a love affair like no other, destined, we believed, to last forever.

There were no warning signs, not a single isolated event to be concerned about beyond the stress and strain of "normal" day-to-day challenges. And yet, Jim and I would both end up in the same hospital at the same time, and both with life threatening illnesses with an uncertain future.

In January 1981, Jim finally got a break, a very big break, when he was offered a senior management position as a community relations officer with Rio Algom Ltd. The major mining company was located in Elliot Lake in Northern Ontario, and we were more than ready to pack up and move on.

With a fond farewell to Nova Scotia, we set off in our two cars, with two kids and two cats, driving almost 2,500 kilometers to Elliot Lake. We decided to drive through the United States because of better winter road conditions. Besides, we wanted to stop in Cape Cod overnight for a visit with Jim's parents. Their unconditional love and financial support had kept our marriage strong while many similar relationships have failed.

In fact, the vast majority of marriages are doomed according to an article, "Managing Bipolar Disorder," in the November 2003 issue of *Psychology Today*: "The condition is still so challenging to tame that 90 per cent of marriages involving a partner with bipolar disorder end in divorce." Other stats in the same article were just as alarming: "Researchers estimate that more than 40 per cent of persons with bipolar disorder abuse alcohol or drugs; 15 to 25 per cent die by suicide, accident, or are killed in altercations triggered in a manic phase."

So far, Jim and I had managed to defy the odds.

Our lives settled into a comfortable routine. We both had high profiles in a community of 17,000 people, because of the nature of our jobs, as well as volunteer work on several committees. I was manager of ELMAR (Elliot Lake Manufacturing and Recycling Ltd.) Company, a major manufacturer of filtration products for the local mining companies. I was also responsible for all of Rio Algom's photography assignments including Jim's bimonthly corporate newsletter, *The Rio Atom*. And I had a weekly column, "As it is" in our local newspaper, *The Standard*. We had many friends and socialized frequently.

For almost ten years, Jim managed to keep his previous medical history private. No one was aware of his psychiatric hospitalizations, not his employer nor his colleagues at work. None of our friends had any inkling of Jim's "misadventures," as he referred to them. Our children were also unaware that their father lived with a genetically transmissible and incurable brain disease, that might put them at risk as well.

Jim had found a doctor, associated with a family clinic at Mount Sinai Hospital in Toronto, who was willing to monitor his blood work and prescribe his medication. Jim paid $88 for a jar of 1,000 lithium capsules at Honest Ed's, a major discount store in Toronto. Jim's moods were stable, and he was also in excellent physical health.

I can't remember Jim taking a day off on sick leave. As far as we were concerned, he was well. Lithium was truly a miracle maintenance drug, without the nasty side effects of antipsychotic medications essential to treat dangerous mood swings that had led to previous hospitalizations.

For the first time in his life, Jim could afford to pursue his passion for fine wines. He invested in wine futures, buying cases of vintage years of French Bordeaux, after the harvest, while the wine was still aging in oak barrels. Jim also purchased a refrigerated wine cellar, large enough to store 150 bottles, to protect his investment. He subscribed to *Wine Spectator* magazine and became an avid collector. His knowledge of wines was astounding, and our friends often sought his advice on best buys.

Elliot Lake was a remarkable community, with high paying jobs, excellent healthcare facilities and plenty of outdoor recreational activities throughout the year. Even though our town had good schools, both English and French, we decided to send Jonathan and Larissa to private boarding schools in Southern Ontario, when they were 12 years old. Jonathan was enrolled at Trinity College School in Port Hope and Larissa went to The Bishop Strachan School in Toronto. We wanted our children to benefit from a wide variety of arts and athletic programs not available in our town. In the summer, Jonathan and Larissa spent a month at the Taylor Statten Camps on Canoe Lake in Algonquin Park in Ontario, Ahmek for boys and Wapomeo for girls. Jim, his sister and mother were all alumni of the camps, where little had changed over the years.

Our major vacation every year, was two weeks in July in Cape Cod, where Jim's parents had a house on the waterfront in Brewster. It was the most marvellous place for all of us to be together, with long walks along the tidal flats during the day and fabulous seafood dinners every night. Although Jonathan and Larissa were away at school most of the year, we were a very close-knit family and cherished the time we spent together, especially when visiting with Jim's parents.

Just as the festive season was approaching, I was conscious of a nagging pain in my lower abdominal area, but I was too busy to see a doctor. I was also feeling a little bloated and concerned about gaining weight, as I looked at myself in the mirror while getting dressed for the company's annual Christmas party.

Not bad for 44, I thought. I was still slim, though my waistline probably reflected too many holiday parties. With a sigh of relief, I managed to slip into my favourite red and blue silk dress, bought at the upscale Saks department store in Boston many years ago. I had a good income so I could afford to splurge occasionally on my wardrobe.

"Are you getting ready?" Jim called out, while I was fixing my hair. He was anxious to get to the rec centre before the guests arrived, more than 200 employees, along with their husbands and wives. The function was his responsibility and everything had to be perfect.

The news earlier in the year that the mining company was in the process of shutting down its operations in Elliot Lake was a major blow for the economy of the town. Many of the company's employees had already left for job opportunities elsewhere. Jim's position was secure for the time being, since Stanleigh Mine would continue to operate until 1996.

Elliot Lake was built in the mid-1950s, largely by the government of the United States that claimed all the uranium reserves in the area to fuel its nuclear weapons program during the Cold War. At peak production, 12 mines were operating in the Serpent River Watershed north of Lake Huron. The American demand was relatively short-lived, leading to several mine closures, until there was renewed interest for the radioactive mineral to fuel the atomic energy industry, not only in Canada, but also in the United States and Japan.

Jim had been under considerable stress in recent months, taking on additional responsibilities, including handling a hotline for queries about the closures. There was no need to worry him about my health concerns, as I popped a couple of Tylenol pills before leaving the house.

We arrived early, so Jim could check on the arrangements to ensure that the bar was fully stocked, and the kitchen was ready to serve refreshments, as soon as guests began to arrive. Dozens of gifts had already been arranged around a large Christmas tree to be handed out by Santa to those holding the lucky ticket, when their number was called.

I was chatting with the DJ as people started to drift in. The pain had subsided, and I was feeling terrific. Jim worked the room, as he always did at these functions, acknowledging everyone's presence and sitting down to chat with some of the old-timers, who had been with the company for more than 25 years. He checked the kitchen regularly and picked up empty beer bottles off the tables.

Whenever I tried to find Jim in the darkened auditorium for a dance, someone else would lead me onto the floor. As always, we were the last to leave and I was exhausted when we finally got home.

The following morning, I woke up in acute pain and told Jim that I was going to the hospital ER. It was Sunday and the doctor's office was closed.

"What for?" he asked.

I mentioned the nagging pain I had been experiencing for several days, but there was no point having him worried as well.

"It's probably nothing," he said, adding, "You have been working too hard and then, you probably spent too much time on the dance floor last night instead of just taking it easy for a change."

Jim was aware of my demanding schedule not only as manager of ELMAR Company, but also as the official photographer for Rio Algom. With the closure of two mines, I was responsible for documenting all the equipment brought to the surface, from dozens of massive jumbo drill rigs, to hundreds of rail cars and portable toilets, either to be sold or safely disposed of, in an environmentally protected landfill.

The waiting room was empty when I arrived at the hospital and I was seen right away. The ER doctor examined me and provided a prescription for the pain. He also set up an appointment for an ultrasound later that week. I left the hospital, picked up my prescription from the pharmacy and drove to the mine site. I spent the rest of the day recording the end of an era, that provided well-paying jobs and exceptional fringe benefits for thousands of miners and their families.

My ultrasound appointment was mid-week. I wasn't worried, not even when the technician called the radiologist to look at the scans of my abdominal area. While I was getting dressed, the nurse advised me that my doctor would see me at 5:30 pm at his office. I hurried back to work. We had a busy production schedule before the plant shutdown for a week during the Christmas holidays.

The medical clinic was quiet when I arrived at the end of the day. The nurse handed me a gown and asked me to get undressed. Then I lay down on the examining table, and felt around my lower abdominal area, but I couldn't figure out what was causing the unrelenting pain.

Dr. David Margetts was old-school English and very conservative in his approach to his patients. That afternoon, however, his voice was gentle and kind after a brief physical examination.

"You are going to require surgery as soon as possible," he said. "You have a mass in your abdomen that needs to be removed."

I looked at him blankly. It was three weeks before Christmas and I hadn't done any shopping.

"How long will I be in the hospital?" I asked.

"I don't know," he said, explaining that he will have to make some calls to find a specialist who will be able to schedule the surgery on such short notice.

When I got home, Jim's face was grim. Dr. Margetts had already called him with the news. Both were members of the Rotary Club and worked together on various fundraising projects. Dr. Margetts didn't pull any punches and advised Jim that my condition was "very grave."

That night, I was woken up by Jim who was sobbing uncontrollably. I tried to assure him that I was going to be alright. I was healthy and strong and would recover from surgery in no time at all. We just held each other for the longest time. Then Jim, fearing the worst, said, "I don't have a picture of you with your short hair."

When I had my hair cut a few months earlier, Jim sulked around the house for days. "You should have asked me first," he said, more than once, making me feel guilty. I am not sure if he ever forgave me, but now he was desperate for a photograph.

I called John Vail first thing in the morning. He was a good friend who had been a professional photographer before retiring to Elliot Lake. I explained that I needed to have a studio portrait taken as soon as possible, without providing any details. The following day, I was sitting in John's makeshift studio in his basement, smiling through an entire roll of film. When I explained the urgency, John stated the obvious: "But you look so healthy." I wasn't surprised with his response, and agreed with him, saying, "I probably am."

In the meantime, Dr. Margetts had located a highly respected oncologist in Toronto, specializing in ovarian cancer, and apparently the best in her field. She had already seen the ultrasound scans and scheduled the surgery for the following week.

The next few days were a blur as I organized our production and delivery schedules. I had a great team working for me so there were no major concerns to deal with during my absence. I also called our main customers and suppliers, advising them I would be taking a few weeks off on sick leave. When I realized that I didn't have a will, I called our company lawyer in Toronto, and he dictated my hand-written will over the phone. I named Jim as the executor of my estate. There was no reason not to appoint him.

We drove to Toronto on a Friday afternoon. We were staying with Jim's parents who had moved into a spacious apartment in Rosedale a few years earlier. I spent all Saturday on a whirlwind shopping expedition for Christmas gifts with Larissa. Otherwise, we spent the rest of the weekend with our closest friends, Lenny and Melissa Finegold. Jim's mood had improved considerably, and I was grateful since I would be counting on his support. We were hoping for the best and had a fabulous time partying late into the night without a care in the world. Or so it seemed.

Jim and I met with Dr. Joan Murphy first thing Monday morning. Her smile was warm and welcoming, putting us at ease at a time when we were both anxious and fearful. Dr. Murphy's examination of my abdominal area was very brief. Only later did I learn that a very large tumour was growing on one of my ovaries and there were other smaller tumours as well. Dr. Murphy advised me to arrive at the hospital early on Wednesday morning for several tests and that surgery was scheduled for the following day. Meanwhile, she put me on a strict liquid diet, essentially chicken broth, Jell-O and apple juice.

"Is it alright to drink wine?" I dared to ask.

"Of course," she said, with an obvious caveat, "as long as it is clear."

Dr. Murphy then asked about our children, and if we were able to make arrangements for them at such short notice. I explained that

Larissa, who was just 14, was at boarding school in the city and Jonathan, 16, was on an exchange program in Japan. For the first time, Dr. Murphy's face showed some concern.

"Is he coming home for Christmas?" she asked.

"No," I responded, explaining that he would not be coming home until the end of the school year which was mid-March.

There was a long pause.

"You may want to consider bringing him home earlier," she suggested kindly, and then quickly added, "Let's wait until after surgery before making the decision. I want to have a better idea of what we are dealing with here."

I was in a daze as we left her office.

"You'll be fine," Jim said, taking my hand and squeezing it. I wasn't so sure. The survival rate for ovarian cancer was very low. Would I see my children graduate from high school, let alone university?

That night, we went to the Senator, a small, intimate restaurant in downtown Toronto's theatre district for a jazz concert. There was nothing on the limited late evening menu that I could have except, perhaps, the French onion soup, if the kitchen was willing to put its house specialty through a strainer.

When the waiter arrived to take the order, Jim's voice was very pronounced as if he was already anticipating an objection.

"French onion soup for the lady, but hold the onions."

The waiter stared at Jim, not sure if he heard him right.

"A bowl of French onion soup without the onions." Jim's voice was now loud enough to carry across the small dining area of the restaurant.

"We can't do that," the waiter replied.

"And why not?" Jim countered, as if it was an ordinary request.

The waiter simply shrugged his shoulders and started to walk away when Jim raised his voice and demanded to see the manager.

I was grateful for the darkness, so I couldn't see the stares of the other diners.

The manager walked over to our table. I was afraid that Jim might create a scene, but the manager just ignored him and quickly diffused the explosive scene with an understanding nod. "Of course, madam."

My bowl of carefully strained French onion soup finally arrived, with a complimentary glass of white wine. That was enough to shut Jim up for the remainder of the evening. When the jazz combo came on, Jim was lost to the music. I finished off the soup and wine and wondered what else to expect.

I was exhausted and fell asleep soon after we arrived back at Jim's parents' apartment. When I woke up in the middle of the night, Jim was still awake, staring at the ceiling.

"Aren't you going to sleep?" I asked.

"I'm just thinking about us," said Jim, assuring me that, "everything will be fine."

I didn't want Jim to know that I was worried about him. His behaviour at the restaurant brought back unwelcome memories of our meal at the Ginger Man in New York almost 20 years ago. Back then, he had been belligerent, creating a scene in the packed restaurant, over a long-forgotten trivial incident. But this is different, I thought. There had not been any signs or symptoms of manic behaviour since we learned the results of the ultrasound the previous week. Besides, Jim had been compliant with his medication. If anything, I thought he was holding up remarkably well considering the circumstances.

We had just sat down in the admitting department of Toronto General Hospital, waiting for my name to be called, when Jim said he recognized a celebrity from a popular television show. He pointed to an old man dressed in baggy pants and wearing a dirty red ski jacket, badly frayed at the cuffs.

"Are you sure?" I asked.

Jim nodded. "Absolutely, I saw him last night on TV."

"You have to be kidding," I responded, taking a closer look at him. "He looks homeless to me."

"Of course, I am sure," said Jim. Now he was angry at me for doubting him as he started to get up from his seat. "Would you feel better if I went over and talked to him?"

"No, no," I said, alarmed at Jim's sudden shift in his mood. "If he doesn't want to be recognized, we should leave him alone."

"So, now you believe me," Jim demanded.

"Of course, I do," I shot back.

What else could I say? We were both obviously under a lot of stress and I let it go. The old man was still sitting there, incognito, or not, reading a tabloid newspaper, when my name was called.

We had no sooner sat down in the admitting clerk's office, when Jim insisted that I have a private room, as specified in his company's insurance policy. It was an ultimatum, not a request.

"Your room will be assigned to you by the nurse on the floor," the clerk informed us, looking at me and ignoring Jim altogether. That wasn't good enough for Jim and he demanded to see her supervisor. In the meantime, I was quickly becoming a nervous wreck. How could Jim be so rude?

When we finally got up to the surgical floor, it was the same scenario all over again.

"My wife is having a private room," Jim insisted, as he approached the nursing station.

"Shhhhhh," the head nurse said, indicating to Jim to be quiet as she quickly escorted us into a private room. No doubt, she had been forewarned that my husband could be difficult if his request was denied.

In any case, I was relieved to have my own room, if for no other reason, but to try to calm Jim down. I kept telling myself that Jim's behaviour was normal for someone who might be anxious about his wife's upcoming surgery with a guarded prognosis.

That morning, I had several scans and didn't arrive back in my room until after the lunch hour. Of course, that didn't matter since I couldn't eat anything. Jim was waiting for me, sitting in a chair by the window, eating a sandwich he had picked up in the hospital cafeteria. Instead of being pleased to see me, Jim was scowling.

"Where the hell were you?" he demanded. "I have been here for hours."

At a time when I most needed his support, I was being chastised for being "late," as if I was on a specific time-table. I attributed Jim's irritability to anxiety and tried to reassure him that I was in good hands. But he was just getting started. Without any provocation, Jim became confrontational, blaming my tumours on my bad behaviour as a "prostitute." Was he referring to the relationships I might have had before we met almost 20 years ago? Even so, Jim had never been the jealous type. Now, as far as he was concerned, I was just a "slut."

I was stunned by his outburst and glared at Jim, not sure how to respond. He was irrational, making wild accusations that had no bearing on my past. At the same time, he was telling me not to worry, softening his voice, when I got up to close the door to my room.

"Lembi, don't you understand that I have total control over everything?"

"Control?" I asked, when I finally caught my breath. "What are you talking about?"

"Lembi, you are just a speck in the universe," Jim explained in a calm, almost soothing voice. "It doesn't really matter whether you recover. I am the only one that matters, because I am 'God.'"

Someone else might have missed the significance of Jim's wild delusional prophecy. Not me. There was no question that he was experiencing a psychotic break with reality and needed to be hospitalized immediately.

I left my room and managed to track down a surgical resident. I could barely control the panic in my voice, when I described my husband's behaviour and my own fears that he might become violent.

I was asked to return to my room and hopefully Jim would not have any reason to leave, while arrangements were being made to hospitalize him.

Ten minutes later, a nurse knocked on the door of my room. My first impression was that she was a very big gal, not someone to mess with. She simply asked Jim if he might come back downstairs, "to sign a few more forms." I could feel Jim tense up for a moment. Was he suspicious?

Jim simply shrugged his shoulders and got up calmly as if everything was perfectly normal. He assumed that the forms were related to my hospitalization and agreed to accompany the nurse, telling me that he would be back soon.

As I walked out into the hall with them, I noticed a male orderly discreetly standing beside a laundry cart near my room. Another male orderly was waiting for the elevator. It was quite evident that the staff was not taking any chances, that Jim might take off. I was left to wonder what was in store for both of us, and for our children, Jonathan and Larissa.

I returned to my room in a state of shock. I unpacked my bag, putting my tape recorder and empty tapes along with the box of pale blue G. Lalo French stationery into the small cupboard. Regardless of my bravado, I was prepared for bad news and would want to write personal notes to family and friends. I put my make-up and toiletries into the drawer. I was determined to look good for visitors and brought a couple of pretty nightgowns to wear when they came to see me. I hung up my colourful Pucci robe that I had bought at an outlet store, during one of our trips to Cape Cod. I figured that I might need a fashion statement to keep up my spirits. Although I was prepared for a lengthy stay, I was expecting Jim to be at my side, holding my hand, and reassuring me that all would be well.

When I couldn't control my tears anymore, I closed the door to my room and lay down on the bed. I cried for the first time in years, not since Jim was hospitalized in California.

A couple of agonizing hours later, my phone rang.

Psych ward

"Hi," said Jim, in a surprisingly cheerful voice. "Guess what?"

"What?"

"You'll never guess where I am calling from?"

I was afraid to ask since Jim sounded elated, as if he had won the lottery. My first thought was that he had managed to convince the staff he was fine, and there was no need to hospitalize him. I would not have been surprised if he was calling me from a nearby bar with a double Scotch in his hand.

Jim didn't miss a beat.

"I'm in the psych ward," he said, laughing. "Can you believe that?"

Although Jim refused to admit that he was ill, he explained that the real reason he agreed to a 72-hour psychiatric assessment was to be close to me. "I'm just upstairs on the eighth floor so I'll be able to visit you whenever I want."

How convenient, was my immediate thought, though I wasn't prepared to see him, not if he was still in a delusional state. And I wasn't sure how to prevent him from visiting me.

"Where is your wallet?" I asked. I was worried that Jim might still take off, if he felt threatened at all.

"It's in a safe," he assured me. "Don't worry about anything. I'll be OK. I have a private room and my own phone. Just take care of yourself. I love you."

"I love you too."

Then I hung up the phone and cried all over again.

Despite Jim's obnoxious behaviour in the admitting office, I was grateful that he had insisted I have a private room. My surgery was scheduled the following morning and I had never felt so alone. I felt betrayed with absolutely no one to blame.

Eventually I called Jim's parents, letting them know that their son was also hospitalized. It was almost too great a burden for anyone to bear with both of us in the hospital, at the same time, requiring urgent medical care. We agreed that Jim had seemed fine that morning, though possibly a little more upbeat than we were. Surely, we had thought, his positive outlook was a good sign.

After years of normal functioning, the sudden shift in Jim's mood and demeanour was all but breathtaking, in its speed and treachery. Once again, Jim managed to maintain a marked degree of control in recent days over his increasing manic behaviour.

I also called Lenny, who came over as soon as he learned that Jim was hospitalized. Like all our friends, he was unaware that Jim had been diagnosed with bipolar disorder almost 20 years earlier. For some reason, Lenny didn't seem surprised, as he described the bizarre transformation of Jim the night before, when they went out for dinner.

"Everything about him was different," he said, talking about someone he had known for ten years, both in corporate and social settings. "It was a total personality change. It was as if the other Jim never existed. He was very animated and working on very high energy levels. Jim was focused on raising a million dollars for a musical and was hoping that I would approach my boss as a major investor in the production. Jim never let up all evening."

When Lenny left, I was alone again. Being hospitalized for cancer surgery was one thing. I had already refused to be haunted by the words in so many obituaries, describing the sad passing of a loved one "after a lengthy courageous battle" with the dreaded disease. With Jim hospitalized as well, instead of sitting at my bedside holding my hand, my resolve was under threat. What I really needed now was to be brave enough to fight another battle and save Jim from the restless enemy deep within his manic mind.

According to his medical report, Jim was "belligerent and loud" and his mood was "labile and unpredictable." There were confrontations with patients and nursing staff soon after he arrived on the ward.

The following morning, while I was in surgery, Jim was being interviewed by the staff psychiatrist, Dr. David Goldbloom. Although he denied being ill, Jim was convinced that there was something sinister in the way Dr. Goldbloom blinked, indicating that he was part of a larger Jewish conspiracy. When Jim grabbed Dr. Goldbloom by the arms in a "threatening manner… showering him with racial slurs," he was declared "dangerous to others and incompetent to consent to treatment." As an "involuntary status" patient, Jim was transferred to the acute care ward accompanied by five male staff members, including Dr. Goldbloom. The medical report describes him as being, "very loud, argumentative and demanding to call his lawyer." At first, Jim refused to take any medication, and then "with firm encouragement," he agreed to take Haldol, in addition to the lithium, to calm him down.

Jim's parents were called to the hospital to sign forms appointing them as substitute decision-makers. They accepted their responsibility without complaint, and without understanding how their son could become so incapacitated, so quickly, and so completely, that he had to be hospitalized against his will. Without a doubt, the emotional stress, or distress, of the possibility of losing me, was the trigger for such a severe psychotic episode.

Jim was furious about the move to a secure ward with its glass-walled cubicles. His street clothes were taken away and he was forced to wear ill-fitting PJs 24/7. The biggest loss was the privileges of a private room and his own phone. When Jim wanted to call me, or anyone else, he had to request permission to use the phone at the nurses' station.

It was just as well. Jim's calls were far from pleasant. In fact, they were very troubling. He was self-absorbed with his own problems and didn't bother to ask me how I was or if I needed anything. Jim resented the fact that our family, friends and colleagues from his company were sending me flowers and get-well cards, when he didn't even rate a fruit basket. A friend, however, picked up a package of cigarettes for Jim at his request and the medical record noted that he was "smoking hourly."

I had never seen Jim smoke before. It's as if the disease had altered his personality, and I was fearful, that it might backfire on him.

One evening, shortly after midnight, Jim demanded the right to call me. Naturally, he was advised that the call would have to wait until the morning. Not to be deterred, Jim grabbed the phone. When the nurse tried to stop him, he grabbed her by the wrist. Then Jim attempted to leave the locked unit to visit me, but the security staff escorted him back to his bed. He was put into a physical four-point restraint, used for volatile patients to restrain both arms and legs. An hour later, a nurse recorded that Jim had freed himself; however, he was sleeping so she left him alone.

During Jim's hospital stay, the medical record noted that he had "little insight into his illness," denying any symptoms of mania. "So, what if I said I was God," he told his nurse. "Maybe it was all theatrics. We all have a bit of God in us."

No matter, Jim was about to appeal his involuntary status. Without consulting me, he hired a lawyer.

Recovery

It was already dark outside when I was brought back to my room after surgery. I had trouble focusing. My body was numb. I couldn't move. My mouth was parched, and I was desperate for something to drink. But I didn't have the strength to summon the nurse, or ask, when she was right beside me, taking my pulse.

For hours, I lay there motionless, drifting in and out of consciousness. Where was Jim when I needed him most? He should be here, beside me, holding my hand. Instead, it was Lenny sitting in the chair, keeping vigil at my bedside.

My next memory was waking up to a sunny day. I could smell an overwhelming scent of flowers, even before opening my eyes. For a moment, I thought I was in a lush garden, as if one of Monet's paintings had come alive. My room was filled with vases of fresh-cut flowers from well-wishers.

The last time I was in a room with so many flowers was at a funeral home during visitation hours when a friend of mine had passed away from colon cancer. I remember seeing the beautiful floral arrangements surrounding her open coffin. We had made plans to get together for lunch not that long ago. Unfortunately, the course of the disease was unrelenting, and then, she was gone. Her eight-year-old daughter was kneeling beside her, praying silently as she fingered her Holy Rosary Beads.

I lay there motionless but I was not in pain. There were tubes everywhere, including up my nose. Suddenly an alarm went off and a nurse rushed in to change the cartridge of my morphine pump. She explained how I could give myself an extra "hit" if I was in pain. And then, I drifted off again.

When I woke up, Dr. Murphy was standing over me, smiling. "I am glad to see that you are recovering so well," she said. Her demeanour quickly changed and the tone of her voice was very serious. "You have had a rough time of it. I have given orders to the nursing staff that you are not to get up for the next 24 hours." Dr. Murphy also mentioned that she had gone to see Jim right after the surgery to let him know that I was in recovery. He had thanked her for the news and seemed to be relieved, though it was apparent to her that he was heavily sedated.

When a nurse came into the room to remove the tubes from my nose, I asked her for a glass of water. She pointed to a hand-written sign taped on the wall behind my bed with "Nothing by mouth" written on it. "Not even a sip?" I pleaded. She shook her head. The sign would stay there for the next three days.

Every time I heard foot steps outside my door, I expected Jim to walk in. Where was he? Why wasn't he here? Dr. Murphy had spoken with him, so he must be OK.

Jim's parents visited that afternoon. In an effort to bolster my mood, his father told me how well I looked. He also asked if I had heard from Jim. When I shook my head, he explained that Jim wasn't able to leave the ward, not after he threatened one of the doctors.

The painful reality began to set in. Jim was seriously ill and there was no pain pump that could alleviate the ache in my gut. I was also scared. When I learned that Jim had tried to leave the locked ward to come and see me in the middle of the night, I knew that the threat of further violent behaviour was very real. What was his mission? Was he coming to comfort me with his healing powers? Or was there another, more insidious motive, such as ensuring the end to my pain by opening the gates of the kingdom of heaven for me?

I let my paranoia get the better of me. But I didn't share my fears with Jim's parents. Surely, they had enough to cope with, with both of us in the hospital for an indeterminate stay. I asked them to let Jim know that I was hoping he would call.

When the phone finally rang, it was Jim. But it was not the call I was expecting. Jim didn't bother to inquire whether I was OK. Instead, he was practically shouting into the phone.

"I want you to get me out of here," he ordered.

When I didn't respond right away, he got nastier, demanding that I also bring him some clothes.

"Clothes?" I asked, not knowing what else to say since Jim was in a very agitated state.

"Yes, don't you get it. They won't let me have my clothes to keep me from going anywhere. I have to wear these dumb PJs that keep falling off me. And they are watching me all the time. I can't take it anymore. You have to get me out of here."

"I'm sorry Jim," I started to apologize, when he interrupted me.

"There's nothing to be sorry about. Just get me out of here. I feel like a caged animal."

Then he hung up the phone.

I felt totally abandoned by the person I loved. How could anyone understand the depth of despair I felt when Jim couldn't care less if I was alive or dead.

When Dr. Murphy came by later in the afternoon, she sat beside me on my bed and smiled.

"You're looking better already," she said.

I didn't feel any better. In fact, I felt much worse because now I was scared. I told her about the phone call with Jim.

"Do you have any reason to be afraid?" she asked.

When I nodded, she suggested that I might want to be moved to another room.

I thought about the offer but decided that sooner or later Jim would find me. He was far too clever to be put off that easily. And I didn't want to aggravate his condition any further. Besides, it would be such an inconvenience for my own family and friends to track me down.

Dr. Murphy then asked me if I was comfortable. I told her I was thirsty and would really like to have a glass of water.

"It will take a few days before the healing begins," she said, explaining that the surgery was very extensive, far more so than she had anticipated. "Until then, I'm sorry that we can't allow anything by mouth."

Just as my circumstances couldn't get any worse, Dr. Murphy provided a glimmer of hope when she said. "The good news is that you don't have ovarian cancer." But that was quickly countered with the dilemma she was facing. "The bad news is that we don't know what you have, except that it is a malignant growth. Quite frankly, I have never seen anything like it before."

For the first time, I was starting to feel sorry for myself. I was too young to die. And then, who was going to look after the children with Jim locked up again, unable to look after himself? That night, I woke up long after midnight and couldn't go back to sleep. I missed Jim terribly. I missed the person I fell in love with and yearned, just to be held in his arms again, and assured that everything would be alright. I worried that lithium would no longer be enough to prevent another major psychotic relapse. I started to cry, quietly at first, and then uncontrollably.

"Is something wrong?" asked the night nurse, when making her rounds.

I started to tell her my story, how my husband was also in the hospital, unable to come and see me. But she interrupted me before I was able to explain why I hadn't been able to see Jim. "The best way to get your mind off your problems," she suggested, "is by turning on your TV." Before I could say anything else, she turned on my TV and left the room, closing the door behind her.

I didn't know what to say. I suppose I was in a state of shock as I stared at the TV screen. There was a movie about ancient Rome with its gladiators fighting in the arena. The nurse was right. The movie was a bore and I soon fell asleep.

Family

Larissa was hugging a small stuffed bear when Lenny brought her to visit me.

"Are you OK Mommy?" she asked quietly, handing over the bear with its bright red Christmas bow.

"I don't look so good, do I?" I responded, though I had put on some make-up and made sure my hair was properly combed.

Larissa sat down beside me and held my hand while I fought back the tears that threatened to overwhelm me. At least I was still alive. And I had to be strong for my children, since Jim was more incapacitated than I was.

"Can I go and see dad?" she asked, barely above a whisper.

Jim had called her earlier that day and she had every right to be confused. Our children were very young when their father had been previously hospitalized and were unaware of his history of mental illness. As far as Larissa could recall, her father had always been well.

I suggested that she wait until the next time she came to visit me. It was a most difficult decision but I was afraid that Jim might frighten her with his complaints about being held against his will. How could I explain to her that our world was falling apart, with both her parents in the hospital, when we had been a "normal" family just two weeks earlier, busy with holiday plans.

Jonathan, on the other hand, was unaware of the drama back home. I was worried whether he would have sufficient supports in Japan to deal with such devastating news, affecting all of us. I also worried about the stigma, a double whammy since the Japanese people are fearful of both conditions, and rarely discuss them privately, let alone publicly. As it was, Jonathan never knew about our hospitalizations until he returned home in mid-March.

My sisters, all younger than me, rallied around my hospital bed. Helen was sitting in the corner of my room when I returned from surgery, knitting a Christmas sweater for her niece. As I drifted in and out of consciousness, I remember being comforted by her presence. My other sisters visited the following day, including Urve, who was eight and a half months pregnant and still drove in from Cleveland with her husband, a doctor. Her twin Vaike offered to stay with me, as long as I needed her. Sarah, the "baby" of the family was also there, lending her support.

My parents, on the other hand, were on a cruise in the Caribbean and were unaware that I had been scheduled for cancer surgery that week. It never occurred to me to spoil their holiday plans. When they came to visit me, instead of being supportive, my mother cautioned me about discussing my "condition" with others, as if such a disclosure might somehow cause her harm.

Jim's parents filled the void. I still treasure the letter from Jim's father, that he wrote after the month he spent with me and the children, during Jim's previous hospitalization in Halifax.

My admiration and love for you knows no bounds and no parent could wish for a better daughter. I am very sincere in this and my feelings go right back to those first days in New York. You have been a wonderful wife and mother… Mom and I have no doubt made many mistakes along the way but I think that we can honestly say we tried to do our best at all times… We are also optimistic about the future and know that you and Jim, together with the children, have many years of happiness ahead. You can always count on our support to the fullest.

Very much love as always, Dad."

Jim's father taught me one of life's most enduring lessons, the importance of unconditional love, even as the destructive force of unpredictable bouts of madness threatened to wreck further havoc in our marriage.

Legal challenges

I was angry. The recurrence of Jim's illness while he was compliant with his meds was a rude awakening for which I was completely unprepared. Jim had responded so well to lithium, for so many years, with all the assurances of a "normal" life. And now, the drug failed him when he needed it the most. It seemed so unfair, considering Jim had never resisted treatment protocols throughout his lengthy hospitalizations. Why should he find himself, all over again, locked up against his will? Just as troublesome was the fact that he refused to acknowledge being severely ill. But that was not surprising.

Anosognosia is a common symptom of psychotic disorders, where individuals have poor insight into the severity of their illness. I was terrified that Jim would take off, if he was released. His credit cards, along with his driver's licence, could once again take him anywhere he chose to go to in Canada and the United States.

There were other concerns as well. Jim's job was on the line. Shortly after he was hospitalized, Jim called a senior vice president at Rio Algom's head office in Toronto for legal advice. After all, the company had a very comprehensive Employee Assistance Program. According to Jim, the vice president was not helpful at all, and hung up on him. Staff who overheard the conversation noted in his medical record their concern that Jim might seriously and irrevocably damage his career.

I also worried about the legal bills. During a phone call, I asked Jim how he was going to pay for the lawyer.

"Don't worry about a thing," he said, rather glibly. "I managed to convince him that I was eligible for legal aid."

"Really?"

If Jim lost his job, my income alone would have disqualified him. But who was I to ask questions? It was painfully evident that Jim could be very convincing, even in the midst of a manic episode. I worried that his incredible control over conflicting emotions could very likely raise doubts about the need to keep him locked up. Jim's application, under the Ontario Mental Health Act, was a request for the Review Board to "inquire into the patient's competency to consent to psychiatric treatment."

I spent the next few days, still hooked up to the morphine pain pump, and barely able to sit up, while meeting with Jim's parents to document their son's history of mental illness. I had requested a legal-size pad of paper (and carbon paper for copies) to provide the lawyer representing the attending physician of the psychiatric ward with as much evidence as possible to keep Jim locked up until he was well enough to leave the hospital. Under no circumstances, should Jim be released from his involuntary status before being stabilized on his medications.

There were the obvious concerns, such as Jim's potential for dangerous actions and violent behaviour. I included other harms as well: the threat to our family's financial security since Jim spends very freely during manic episodes, racking up significant debts on a number of credit cards; the threat to his current and future career prospects for a responsible management position in a major corporation; and the threat to his relations with family and friends, who have never seen Jim in a manic state, another persona altogether, someone who is irritable, angry, often confrontational, and at times hostile and antagonistic.

Jim dressed appropriately for the hearing, held on December 21, wearing grey flannel slacks, a navy blazer, a pale blue shirt and a red silk tie. He was not your image of someone labelled by others as "crazy," who needed to be locked up against his will. The decision issued the following day, revoked his involuntary status. Jim had been able to convince the Review Board that he possessed "sufficient control so as to prevent matters from getting totally out of hand." According to the ruling, "Mr. Buchanan clearly has a profound understanding of his condition. Unfortunately, he is not willing to acknowledge the severity of his current situation."

Although Jim had engaged in minor assaults while on the ward, apparently there was "no compelling evidence which demonstrated a likelihood of serious bodily harm to others." The fact that Jim had been violent with me was "not an issue at the moment for the simple reason that she is hospitalized and will continue to be in the hospital for some time."

Despite the revocation of his involuntary status, Jim was "strongly encouraged" to stay put. "The evidence heard by the Board leaves little doubt that Mr. Buchanan's best interest is to remain in the hospital at this time. There can be no doubt that discharge at this time will result in serious risk to Mr. Buchanan's career, finances and family stability."

Fortunately, Jim had been compliant with the medication regimen prescribed by his doctor. By the time the Board's decision was issued, Jim was "well enough" to understand that he still required hospital care until his medical condition was fully stabilized.

Jim was able to get an overnight pass to spend Christmas at his parents' home. I had already been discharged to their care a few days earlier. As much as I was grateful for a new lease on life, it was not a happy time. I had not mentioned anything to Jim about the financial catastrophe facing us. That had to wait. I still wanted to salvage as much holiday joy as possible.

We spent a traditional Estonian Christmas Eve at my parents' home and Christmas Day with Jim's family. As always, Jim's parents were generous with their cash gifts. I decided to set aside the funds for emergencies that might arise with the children. Jim planned to buy an expensive new watch for himself. It was quite evident that he was still experiencing signs of mild mania, or hypomania as it is otherwise known, since he was focused on spending his money on something he didn't need and certainly couldn't afford. The fact that he was deeply in debt would have never occurred to him.

Financial chaos

While I was in the hospital, I was startled by the sheer size of the Xpresspost envelope delivered to me one afternoon. Jim had always been very secretive about his finances and used a P.O. Box for his personal mail. Our next-door neighbour worked for the post office and kindly sent me the mail that had piled up during our absence. Most of the mail was credit card statements. The number of banks represented in the pile spread out on my bed was mind boggling.

Although I had no right to do so, I opened Jim's mail. I was stunned to find that many of the credit cards were already maxed out. It appeared that he was only making minimum monthly payments and much of it was interest. I was afraid to add up the total and just shoved his mail back into the envelope. I sat there for a long time, completely bewildered by such a shocking discovery.

How could his spending have gotten out of control when Jim was earning a good income? I blamed myself. I should have been paying more attention to his purchases, especially when he ordered several cases of expensive French wines. Our travel budgets and restaurant tabs were probably excessive as well. But then, our cost of living in Elliot Lake was relatively low. In any case, if I would have raised my concerns, Jim would have just ignored them. Money management had been a sore point almost from the beginning of our relationship and had threatened our marriage more than once.

It became very clear that I couldn't trust Jim to be the executor of my estate. In addition to the house in Nova Scotia, I had business interests in Elliot Lake. With both children attending private school, I needed to protect their interests as well, if I became a cancer statistic. I called our firm's lawyer, who arranged for a colleague to come to the hospital and draw up a new will for me.

Unfortunately, there was no easy fix for the financial predicament facing us when we returned home. The total tab for 14 credit cards exceeded $65,000. I had no choice but to mortgage my house in Nova Scotia to cover the debt. Jim reluctantly handed over his credit cards. I cut them up and threw them out.

It was snowing on January 6, when we left Toronto for Elliot Lake. Jim was still heavily medicated and unable to drive. After a gruelling four-hour drive, we stopped at the Swiss Chalet in Parry Sound for lunch. Jim threatened to walk out because the restaurant was serving frozen rather than fresh cut fries. I didn't care. I needed a break.

By the time we got home that night, I was exhausted emotionally and physically. I was angry at Jim for making my life so miserable. I was angry because I believed that he was discharged too early, before he was fully stable on his meds. I was angry at myself for not being stronger in the midst of adversity. Surely other families coped better under similar circumstances.

My meeting with Dr. Murphy went well enough. The pathology results indicated that I had a very rare form of uterine cancer, endometrial stromal sarcoma. As a palliative measure, I was prescribed large doses of a common hormonal drug that had some promise, as far as preventing further tumour growth. Just the same, Dr. Murphy noted in her letter to Dr. Margetts that, "She is still at risk for a poor outcome and ultimate death from this disease."

The prognosis for Jim was also guarded. Now that the mania had subsided, Jim was severely depressed. Back then, there were limited choices in the medicine cabinet for someone like Jim, always at risk of another manic episode with devastating consequences. Although he continued to be compliant with his medications, they failed to rescue him from the depths of depression. When his body no longer tolerated the assault of powerful antipsychotic drugs, they were discontinued, and the risk of suicide became a major concern.

After Jim's wife left him in November 1971, he had written a lengthy suicide note, which he shared with me soon after we met. Thankfully, Jim had shelved the letter for another day that never materialized:

My life has been a series of misadventures. I wish I could look forward to a bright future – but unfortunately, I don't see it. The happiest days of my life turned into a nightmare... I thought I was on the road to some measure of success... Deceived again... I have gone through hell. I see no future for myself... I am lost, and alone...

When one contemplates suicide, one searches for the answers to many questions. Obviously, one asks why? What for? Isn't life ultimately worth living? How can one say he is defeated at twenty-six? The answers are not easy. The basic answer is that one feels the futility of it all. The negatives outweigh the positives… and the anxiety isn't worth it.

There was every reason to worry when Jim's condition continued to deteriorate. Unable to return to work due to persistent disabling symptoms of bipolar disorder, Jim had been eligible for short-term disability payments, paid by Rio Algom. As a result, he received his full salary for six months, from the date of his hospitalization on December 13, 1990.

In early spring, Jim's employer dismissed him despite the fact that he was still on medical leave authorized by his doctor. Jim's self-esteem plummeted to a new low and he became obsessed with his failures. These feelings were exacerbated when his application to the Prudential Insurance Company of America for long-term disability (LTD) benefits was denied. There was also the fight to access Canada Pension Plan (CPP) disability benefits and the Disability Tax Credit (DTC) when these applications were initially rejected.

More than anything else, Jim just wanted his life back.

In the referral to the Mood Disorders Clinic at The Clarke Institute of Psychiatry, Dr. Margetts had asked for an assessment of the "severity of Jim's bipolar disorder," noting that he was having "difficulty coping with the easiest of tasks."

In a letter dated November 23, 1992, after meeting with Jim, Dr. Robert Cooke addressed why Jim was having problems with his claim for disability benefits:

Interestingly, while Mr. Buchanan implied that he is entitled to a disability pension because of manic-depressive illness, he denied specific symptoms of mania or depression over the past two years since his discharge from the Toronto General Hospital… Despite Mr. Buchanan's protestations to the contrary, it is possible that he is suffering from the depressive phase of bipolar illness… Although he denies a specific depressed mood, he has anxiety, impaired concentration and social withdrawal.

Dr. Cooke also arranged for a series of psychological tests in January 1993 to help determine Jim's prospects as far as finding a meaningful and rewarding job that would restore his sense of self-esteem. The results of two days of intensive testing were crushing because of persistent deficits in social and occupational functioning. His potential for vocational rehabilitation would "be contingent on stabilizing his current psychological state."

The test showed performance characterized by slow response times and a focus on imperfection as well as inappropriate social and verbal judgment, hostile defensive responses, a disjointed quality and possibly compromised judgment... In summary, Mr. Buchanan is currently experiencing a significant degree of distress which manifests itself in the form of high levels of emotionality... it is evident that Mr. Buchanan is suffering from a poorly controlled bipolar affective disorder.

In May 1993, Jim finally received confirmation from the federal government that he was entitled to CPP disability payments retroactive to June 1991, including interest. The good news was that both children were also eligible for a monthly allowance of $113 while they were still in school. Accessing the DTC was more complicated and would take longer.

The next ten years were pivotal as far as legal battles to secure the income supports to which Jim was entitled not just from Prudential but also from the federal government. Severe mental illness was not viewed as disabling as many physical impairments, largely because the signs and symptoms are not always present, although the effects of the impairment are challenging most of the time.

Chapter Five - Double Jeopardy

Another nightmare

In June 1993, I suffered a setback and ended up back at Toronto General Hospital. I worried about Jim, and whether my hospitalization would trigger another manic episode. And yet, he seemed to be fine. While I was undergoing tests, Jim visited me daily, brought flowers and was very supportive – a sharp contrast from my previous hospitalization in December 1990. My room-mate thought Jim was very charming and made a point of telling me that I was fortunate to have such a caring husband.

It was just as well that Jim wasn't worried about me. The last couple of years had been very difficult because of Jim's low mood and deep-rooted anxieties. We were faced with the realization that recovery from recurrent episodes of elevated mood followed by periods of debilitating depression was more difficult and would take longer.

Not long after being discharged from the hospital in January 1991, Jim started to develop disturbing side effects that were common with a first-generation antipsychotic medication, such as Haldol, which he continued to take in low doses in addition to lithium. His hands trembled. He was also suffering from akathisia which is sometimes referred to as the "rabbit syndrome" because he couldn't sit still for any length of time. Even more troubling was Jim's lack of control over facial muscles and the continuous chewing motion. Despite the increased risk of a recurrence of mania, Haldol was discontinued since the condition, known as tardive dyskinesia, could be permanent. Fortunately, the side effects slowly diminished and eventually disappeared.

Although I was back in the hospital in June, it was encouraging to see Jim's disposition greatly improved. He was happy to be back in Toronto, since the city was "far more stimulating" than Elliot Lake. Jim not only managed to get a couple of tickets to the musical *Miss Saigon* which had just opened in Toronto, but he also convinced my doctor to let me out on an evening pass. On other evenings, Jim was going out for dinner with family and friends.

Jonathan, who had just graduated from high school, happened to mention that they were dining at expensive restaurants and dad was ordering pricey wines. When I mentioned this to Jim, he just shrugged off my concerns and assured me that others were helping to pick up the tab. Jim was always able to rationalize his actions, regardless of his state of mind. I had been caught in that trap before. Why did I not see it then?

Just as disconcerting was the call from Larissa one afternoon after she and Jim had gone shopping at Sporting Life. Apparently, he had spent more than $200 for five shirts as well as a jacket for himself but refused to pay for the $10 boxer shorts she wanted. Larissa was distraught since her father had always been very generous and she couldn't understand why he was suddenly being "so stingy."

Under any other circumstances, I would not have been alarmed. But Jim never had the patience to shop for clothes, let alone buy five shirts for himself. And then to deny such a small request from his daughter. There was no doubt in my mind. Jim was on a spending spree characteristic of uncontrolled manic behaviour. I was worried enough to contact Dr. Cooke on Friday morning, as I was waiting to be discharged. I expressed my concern whether the purchase of five shirts warranted serious discussion of manic spending. Dr. Cooke agreed, and acknowledged that Jim might require hospitalization if he continued to exhibit unusual behaviour.

On Saturday night, Jim and I went out for Chinese food with our friends Lenny and Melissa. We had every reason to celebrate since I was given a clean bill of health with no evidence of new tumour growth. It also appeared that Jim had turned the corner as well, though I thought it was odd he was wearing his jeans. I couldn't recall Jim ever being dressed so casually when going out for dinner. Even if I were to make the association of Jim wearing the same pair of jeans during his previous manic episodes, what would it prove? Jim seemed to be fine, and we were enjoying an evening out with our friends.

On Sunday, we had a pleasant lunch with my family and Jim was more complimentary toward my mother than usual. Rather than being concerned, I was relieved that they were getting along so well. Later, in the afternoon, we drove out to Mississauga for a dinner party at a former mine manager's home. It was a lovely day and I was so very grateful, not just for the assurances from Dr. Murphy that my cancer was in remission but also the knowledge that Jim had bounced back to his old self. All I could think of at that moment was how lucky I was, when true love really is forever.

We were chatting about nothing in particular during the drive when Jim mentioned that his mother probably knew a number of potential investors. It was as if lightning struck, and I immediately tensed up.

"Investors? For what?" I inquired, trying to be as casual as possible.

"I've been thinking again," he said, suddenly excited and energetic, "about producing that musical we talked about when we still lived in New York."

There was a vague recollection that Jim may have talked about producing his own musical, when we met 20 years ago. And that was when he was beginning to exhibit signs of grandiose behaviour.

Suddenly, I became very frightened. There was no doubt in my mind that Jim needed to be hospitalized. However, I couldn't let him know that I suspected he was seriously ill. As soon as we reached our friends' home, I alerted them of my suspicions. Jim and Ann agreed to help me take him to The Clarke later that evening. While everyone was enjoying drinks and appetizers, I was in the basement office calling the hospital to arrange for Jim to be admitted. Dr. Cooke had already alerted the ER staff of the possibility that he might need urgent medical intervention, even if he refused to acknowledge that he was ill.

During dinner, Jim was very sociable and entertained everyone with his extensive knowledge of wines. He had brought a bottle of Chardonnay from the Roxburgh vineyards in Australia, our hosts namesake. There was never a moment that anyone would have questioned Jim's behaviour as anything except "normal." I was amazed at his extraordinary control over his emotions and wondered if I was overreacting. Jim wasn't exhibiting any of the common symptoms of manic behaviour. He was as "cool, calm and collected" as I had ever seen him.

After dinner, Jim was still in good spirits and agreed to be driven to The Clarke, perhaps just to humour me. However, as soon as he realized that the door to the ER was locked behind him, Jim panicked, insisting that he wasn't ill. Once the resident psychiatrist started to ask questions, Jim's mood suddenly shifted; he became combative, threatening to "take everything to the press."

The admission report indicated that Jim was in a "manic state anxious, irritable and hostile, exhibiting grandiose beliefs and impaired judgment and insight." In addition to the lithium he was already taking, Jim was prescribed Haldol, despite the risk of permanent, harmful side effects. There really was no other choice since acute manic symptoms must be controlled as soon as possible or the patient's condition may continue to deteriorate.

Jim was admitted to the crisis unit as a voluntary but certifiable patient. I learned later that Jim was confined to his room and put under continuous observation. A social worker captured the severity of his mental state with the following notation in his medical record: "He refused to let me contact anyone in his family saying that he could not prevent me from doing so, but I would be doing so at the risk of my death."

Jonathan and I visited Jim the following morning before returning to Elliot Lake. He was sitting in the common room with a female patient and listening intently as she described her own paranoid symptoms. When she called him "doctor," I realized that she thought Jim was one of the staff psychiatrists.

"And what are you so afraid of?" he asked her gently, making notes on an advertising card he had pulled out of a magazine.

"Rats," she responded with the look of real terror in her eyes. "They are all over my house."

"Then, why don't you get a cat." suggested Jim.

"Why would I want a cat?"

"To get rid of the rats."

Outwardly, Jim was calm and relaxed. I suspected the opposite since he had shaved off his beard for the first time in 15 years. While Jonathan was somewhat startled by his father's new image, I was horrified by Jim's impulsive action to alter his appearance so drastically. I couldn't help wondering if there was a particular message he was trying to convey.

Were we wrong to leave Jim behind? There were no outward signs of manic behaviour he exhibited the previous evening. Indeed, Jim seemed to be resigned to staying at the hospital for the time being, confident that he would be able to go home soon. He walked us to the elevator and thanked us for coming to visit him.

When Jonathan and I arrived home that evening, I listened to the messages on our answering machine. The salesman from Grand Touring Automobiles in Toronto had called several times about a missed appointment that morning. I returned his call, letting him know that Jim wouldn't be coming in. When he provided the details of the sale of a used Jaguar, I explained that Jim had been hospitalized at The Clarke.

"No kidding," he said. There was a long pause before he continued. "You may not know but we get a lot of kooks coming in here. I can spot them, the moment they come in the door, but not your husband. No way. He knew exactly what he wanted to buy and how to negotiate. He also knew that he could probably get a better deal from the bank to finance the purchase than what we could offer him."

Apparently, Jim had put a $1,000 down payment on his American Express card. He had essentially traded in our beloved "Beast," a four-wheel-drive Toyota Land Cruiser, by handing over the vehicle registration as a goodwill gesture until Monday, when he expected to complete the financing details for the Jaguar. Later, when I asked Jim why he didn't opt for a Ferrari or a Maserati in the luxury car showroom, he remarked casually, "One has to be reasonable. I didn't have access to $250,000."

A few days after Jim was hospitalized, a nurse called and informed me that she had over-heard him on the pay phone booking a family vacation to Walt Disney World for that weekend. When I called Jim, he was very excited about the trip and gave me the confirmation number for two nights stay at the Comfort Inn in Orlando and other details so I could make the final arrangements and book the air travel. Instead, I canceled the trip. I also canceled his phone card.

I always suspected that Jim had replaced most of the credit cards I had cut up, when I bailed him out two years ago. Granted, I had no authority to cancel his credit cards. Still, I worried that Jim had the means to take off again in a manic state as he had previously done with his trip to California in 1978. I simply called each bank from my old list and advised them that my husband had lost his wallet, but he was too embarrassed to call himself. Could they please cancel the current credit card and issue a replacement?

I was just getting started.

A drug and a curse

Our financial situation was dire. I was meeting with bankers and lawyers. There was little I could do without Jim's co-operation. In fact, he never expressed any interest in my concerns. For that reason, I was no longer as forgiving as I once was, leaving me more vulnerable to increased hostility, and possibly violence, if he did not recover sufficiently from his current manic state.

While one of the most common sources of conflict among couples is money, I tried to steer clear of these discussions as much as possible. Early on, I knew that arguing over finances would eventually destroy our marriage since our views about saving and spending were poles apart. The groundwork was already set in Nova Scotia, where we established separate bank accounts. As long as Jim was working, or had access to severance and pension income, he paid for most of the household expenses. I took care of my personal needs, as well as those of the children. When they went to private school, I picked up the tab. We usually shared travel expenses.

Jim's father was also losing patience when he learned that Jim had racked up another $15,000 on credit cards. He was shocked to learn that I had personally bailed out Jim two years earlier, when the total tab exceeded $65,000.

Truth be told, I had been too embarrassed at the time to let his father know what a mess we were in, and admit that I had no idea that Jim had gone back on his word and asked the banks to reissue his credit cards.

I suspected that some of the debt was sitting in his climate-controlled wine cellar in our basement, which Jim kept locked. It wasn't until I got home, found the key and discovered that the cellar was full, holding approximately 150 bottles. A receipt from LCBO (Liquor Control Board of Ontario), stuck to one of the bottles and dated August 31, 1992, provided a clue: 12 bottles of Chardonnay from Chalk Hill wineries in California for $203.40; three bottles of C.S. 87 Spec. Sel. for $231.60.

Some of the wines Jim had purchased turned out to be extremely good investments. Not that he could have sold a bottle of 1982 Chateau Margeaux valued in excess of $1,000 to a restauranteur to help pay some bills. Over the years, however, Jim managed to benefit financially by donating a select number of his prized French vintages for their appraised value to the Canadian Opera Company's wine auctions to reduce his taxes under CRA's strict rules regarding charitable donations.

It wasn't enough to avoid another credit card crisis.

I was deeply hurt by Jim's dishonesty regarding his compromised financial position. How could he keep filling his cellar with expensive bottles of wine when I was struggling to keep the children in private school? And yet, Jim had no interest in trying to justify any of his purchases. Besides, he made a point of telling me that conversations about money made him "tense." I reminded him that he had created the crisis and I was pretty darned anxious as well.

As Jim's father indicates in his letter, we were both, once again, caught up in the twilight zone of uncertainty and despair.

The story you relate seems quite unbelievable but of course we know it is not. And we are much more concerned about you and the situation you find yourself in, than we are in Jim, who just seems to come out of these "episodes" as if nothing had ever happened, and it was just a bad dream. In the meantime, the full brunt of the problem falls on you.

Credit cards are nothing but a drug and a curse... After the New York "episode," I thought we agreed to get rid of them for good... You say in your letter, "I am not sure I can put up with Jim's need for credit cards anymore." In our opinion, you must not agree to any need... We do realize that this is easier said than done...

We know you love him very much or you would not have endured such pain and grief over the years. We are sure that anyone else would have walked out on him many years ago. We trust that Jim loves you in the same manner but he certainly has a very strange way of showing it.

A few days later, another letter arrived from Jim's father with a substantial cheque to assist with some of my "immediate problems." I was extremely grateful to be on the receiving end of his parents' goodwill when he wrote: "There is no need for you to pay all or part of it in the near future. Let's get some of the smoke cleared before we even think of that."

The remainder of his letter was very serious, with the warning: "Something drastic has to be done." Not surprisingly, Jim's father refused to bail out his son's current credit card debt and threatened to cut him out of his will unless Jim relinquished control over his financial affairs to me.

Such a move was not as simple as it might sound.

I investigated whether Jim could be declared mentally incompetent by a judge, who could then appoint me to look after his financial affairs. While it was possible, I was advised that it would be a costly venture, at least $3,500 for the documentation and legal fees. And Jim, once he "recovered," could go back to court and, in all likelihood, convince the judge that he was now capable of looking after his own affairs. The court order would be rescinded, and I would be no further ahead.

I could not have been more discouraged by the revelation that there was no practical legal recourse to protect our family assets from a bipolar spouse with impulsive spending habits and impaired judgment. Instead of street drugs, Jim was seduced by the endless possibilities offered by credit cards and simply could not live without them. He needed them to ease the anguish of his depressed mood and he needed them just as much, if not more, to fuel the endless possibilities of his manic mind.

Just the same, I was desperate. At the hospital discharge meeting with his psychiatrist and social worker, I needed to set some ground rules. Financial control was always a sore subject for Jim, but he eventually agreed to have his income deposited into a joint bank account, now that he was receiving CPP disability benefits. At the very least, I could start paying down some of his current debt.

Admittedly, our living expenses in Elliot Lake were minimal. I still had to set aside funds for Jonathan, who was going to the University of British Columbia in Vancouver in September and Larissa, who was returning to boarding school in Toronto. When it was obvious in January 1991 that Jim was unable to return to work, I wrote to the children's schools about our inability to meet their tuition and boarding expenses. They were excellent students and both schools were very generous with their financial aid packages.

I also put my house in Nova Scotia up for sale. I simply couldn't afford the $800 monthly payments for the mortgage when I bailed Jim out from his previous credit card debt. I had hoped that he would have received his long-term disability payments from Prudential, which would certainly ease the cash crunch. Although Jim's lawyer had filed a claim in court against the insurer, we still didn't have a trial date to fall back on, and no guarantees.

When Jim was released on July 19, his doctors felt that he was still at a high risk for a subsequent manic or depressive relapse. At home, he continued to take Haldol at a decreased dosage. Even so, Jim complained that he felt like a zombie. His tremors persisted and he had trouble sleeping at night.

Larissa was back at camp working as a counsellor. Jim thought that Jonathan, who was 19, should be working as well, while I was grateful that he was home for the summer.

I was determined to maintain an active social life, inviting friends for dinner on a regular basis. After all, we had a well-stocked wine cellar, although the Bordeaux first growth vintages would not be ready for drinking for another ten years. Jonathan was a terrific sous chef and a very capable dishwasher. Besides, Jim always perked up when friends visited. It was as if there was a spark that was easily ignited from within, whenever someone dropped by the house. I couldn't understand how Jim's mood could shift from sad to glad so easily. How could he be practically paralyzed by his depressed mood during the day and manage to act reasonably upbeat, indeed, "normal" in the evening when company arrived at our doorstep? I wondered if our friends thought that Jim was a fraud, collecting disability benefits when he appeared to be well?

At the end of August, the three of us piled into the Land Cruiser with Jonathan's belongings for the 3,800-km trip to Vancouver. Jim was unable to drive because he was still taking powerful psychotropic drugs. Although Jonathan had his license, and was a careful driver, Jim became anxious with him behind the wheel, threatening to get out at the next stop light. Whenever Jim was anxious, I watched him like a hawk for further signs and symptoms that might lead to another manic episode. I have never been a good long-distance driver but I persevered. There was no other choice.

I made an effort to find lodgings for the evening by five o'clock, so we could relax during dinner and get a good night's sleep. One afternoon, while driving through the prairies, in the middle of nowhere, Jim advised me that it was almost five o'clock and he needed to take his medications. Jonathan checked the map and noted that the next town was still an hour away. That's when Jim began to panic. It's hard to fathom how vulnerable he was at the time, living with the fear that if he deviated from a strict schedule, he might experience another relapse. There were other irritants as well.

Jim wasn't pleased that I was keeping an eye out for reasonably priced accommodations when we arrived at our destination each day. He fretted about the condition of the mattresses in so-called "cheap" motels, so I had to check out not only the room but also the bed to prevent him from complaining.

We spent a few days with friends in Vancouver before heading back home. Now that there was just the two of us, we decided to take a leisurely route through the northern United States, including a detour to visit Yellowstone National Park in Montana and the Badlands in South Dakota. I had noticed before that travel acted as an elixir for Jim; he was more relaxed and his mood steadily improved.

We were also pinning our hopes on an innovative treatment for bipolar disorder since lithium therapy, on its own, could no longer ward off another devastating manic episode. In September, Jim was prescribed Epival (divalproate sodium) an anti-convulsant drug that had been in use since 1984 to control certain types of seizures by preventing excessive electrical activity in the brain. Its use as a mood stabilizer was a more recent development when a doctor treating his patients with epilepsy noticed that their temperament improved while taking the medication.

In November, however, Jim became severely depressed. I was afraid that he might be suicidal and worried about him whenever I left for work in the morning. Dr. Cooke recommended a short-term trial with 50 mg Zoloft (sertraline HCI), an anti-depressant, hoping that the presence of both mood stabilizers, lithium and Epival, would protect him from a drug-induced mania. We were aware of the risks, but we were also desperate for relief of the black clouds that persisted overhead, day after day, and week after week.

Jim remembers a pleasant, heady feeling, being very light on his feet, as if he was floating on air. I remember that he accused me of trying to poison him. There was no choice but to stop taking the anti-depressant. Not surprisingly, Jim slipped back into the deep hole of despair. In a letter, dated December 6, 1993, Dr. Cooke's overall prognosis for Jim was poor.

In summary, Mr. Buchanan has continued to have fairly persistent and fluctuation in the symptoms of his illness complicated by medication side-effects which had disabled him from his usual occupation... This tends to strengthen my opinion that he has a very refractory illness which does not respond well to usual treatments for this condition and which very likely was continuously disabling during the past two to three years.

Just the same, we were cautiously optimistic about better days in the New Year.

Part III

Legal Challenges

Chapter Six – Financial Security

Promises, promises

Picking a fight with the Prudential Insurance Company of America had us wading into uncharted territory, with no precedent to guide us. Instead of continuing with monthly disability payments where Rio Algom left off in June 1991, the country's largest insurer kept dragging its feet, asking for detailed information related to Jim's job description as well as additional medical reports. At the end of the day, all efforts to comply with numerous requests were futile. In a letter dated September 14, 1992, Prudential denied Jim's claim, stating, "We do not have medical information to support you being Totally Disabled for your occupation as of June 13, 1991."

Of course, Prudential was fully aware of the severity of Jim's medical condition from the outset and authorized Rio Algom to pay short-term disability benefits for six months based on the information provided by Jim's physician, Dr. Margetts. However, when it was Prudential's turn to pay, the company refused to pick up the tab. Without providing an explanation, Prudential brushed off his medical opinion as irrelevant.

We ran into similar roadblocks trying to access federal income security programs. Despite letters from Dr. Margetts requesting "utmost urgency" in the review of Jim's applications due to his deteriorating mental health, it took two years to receive monthly CPP disability benefits and three years to claim the DTC. Dr. Margetts noted that the "anxiety resulting from his financial situation has had a very adverse effect on his mental state… His manic-depressive state has become much worse despite the fact that he has continued to take his medication."

While Prudential was still reviewing his file, Jim lost patience and complained to the Ontario Insurance Commission. When he was advised that his "only recourse was through the courts," I met with

131

Doug Kearns, an Elliot Lake lawyer with a general practice that included the manufacturing sector in our town.

Mr. Kearns filed the Statement of Claim on November 4, 1992, with the Ontario Superior Court of Justice in Sault Ste. Marie. He was aware that insurers had largely been able to avoid major payouts for disability claims that involved a mental illness. Nevertheless, he was confident Jim had a strong case. It could also be an important win for a small-town lawyer, setting a precedent for people sidelined from their jobs because of mental disabilities. The company's insurance policy for senior staff left the door wide open with the proviso that the employee was required to be "totally disabled, by reason of accidental bodily injury or illness, to perform the substantial and material duties of his own occupation." The question was whether Jim met the legal requirement during the six months following the onset of his psychosis in December 1990.

The problem, quite simply, was the lack of substantive corroborating medical evidence to satisfy Prudential, when trying to assess the disabling effects of bipolar disorder. Although Jim did not have to be completely incapacitated to qualify for LTD benefits, he still had to prove that he was unable to do his job. In a court document filed by Mr. Kearns, he provided an explanation why it was so difficult for medical practitioners to accurately evaluate the severity of Jim's mental illness:

The manic nature of Mr. Buchanan's disease makes him believe that he is fine, in fact, much more than fine, superior. His disease makes it difficult for him to admit that he has an illness... Admission of mental health problems carries a social stigma and embarrassment not associated with other diseases... Mr. Buchanan was very frightened by this manic episode. It was the first one he had suffered while continuing his medication. Up until this incident, his illness had been controlled by lithium. It was now out of control. Drawing attention to this mental illness left Mr. Buchanan, at least in his mind, at the mercy of doctors, who had the power to essentially imprison him in hospital, as had happened in December 1990 and in the summer of 1993.

The Statement of Claim included monthly payments for long-term disability, a declaration at trial that Jim continued to be "totally disabled" within the terms of the policy, costs and $200,000 in punitive damages as per notation #7 in the claim:

Despite being provided by the Plaintiff with medical and other proof required, the Defendant has refused to pay, in full knowledge that such refusal exacerbates the Plaintiff's mental illness and continues his totally disability... he is entitled to punitive damages to compensate him for the Defendant's willful refusal to abide by the terms of the policy.

Prudential made a counter-offer of $25,000.

It was an insult.

We knew that a trial would be very stressful for both of us. There was a lot at stake, more than half a million dollars, if Jim met the eligibility criteria for the next 20 years. It would take two more years to secure a trial date.

In the meantime, we were both dealing with major health issues as well as financial concerns.

The following spring, I was back in Toronto for a routine check-up. There was the nagging question of further tumour growth, when an ultrasound raised some concerns. Dr. Murphy was mindful of the grim reality facing us, that my hospitalization for additional tests might trigger yet another manic episode, sending Jim back to the hospital as well. We decided on a more conservative approach, to continue with my medication regimen, and postpone further investigations unless I was having specific symptoms that needed to be addressed. I made the decision not to share any of the information with Jim, except to say that I was fine and wouldn't need any more tests for a while.

Besides, I was worried about Jim's erratic behaviour. I continued to be faced with the conundrum of the disease that took such a hold over Jim despite advancements in medications and innovative treatment protocols. He was increasingly preoccupied with his own problems and failed to recognize that I was suffering silently over my own indeterminate future health and well-being. Nor did Jim understand how stressful it was living with a bipolar partner. When we argued, I was always on the defensive, feeling guilty about my emotional outbursts. It was as if I was the one who was unreasonable and unrealistic as I struggled with our deteriorating relationship. Sometimes, I questioned my own sanity.

I could not have been happier when Jonathan came home from university in May for the summer holidays. I hate to admit it, but I needed his unwavering support to keep me on an even keel. However, Jim wasn't happy with Jonathan at home, complaining that we couldn't afford to feed him. I reminded Jim that I was paying the bills, including the mortgage on the house registered in his name.

In fact, I was digging my own hole, accumulating significant debt to keep Larissa in private school, as well as paying for Jonathan's post-secondary education. That's when Jim decided to renege on my access to his CPP disability benefits, saying that the decision to give up control over his financial affairs last summer was made under duress. He was furious because I was using "his" money to pay down "his" credit card debt.

When Jim threatened to lock me out of our home, I asked him to transfer the deed for the house into my name. I was worried about losing the house, if Jim was forced to declare bankruptcy since he refused to cancel his credit cards, or at the very least, surrender them to me for safekeeping. When Jim refused to transfer the house to me, we were at an impasse. I was emotionally drained and just plain frustrated. I was beginning to dislike the person I had become and hating Jim for causing so much pain and suffering in our lives.

I decided that the ownership of the house was non-negotiable and moved in with friends. Perhaps it wasn't the best way of handling the current crisis, though I couldn't think of any other options. I was also being terribly unfair to Jonathan, expecting him to keep an eye on his father despite the tensions between the two of them.

At the time, Jim and I were already seeing a psychiatric social worker, Pam Sargent Hamer, to try to resolve some of our differences and salvage our marriage. I expressed my sentiments in a fax to her:

Just to let you know, I left Jim (temporarily) last night and I'm staying with friends. As I was leaving, Jim promised that I could have total financial control. The promise was more out of desperation than anything else. I really don't know how I can trust him anymore… His history (when "well"), is one of manipulation of financial matters. Of course, Jim justifies everything. But, too often, his judgment is screwed up.

The major problem, beyond the financial issues, is the fact that Jim feels cornered, trapped. I don't know whether I can continue to live with someone who blames me, rather than himself, for this predicament. I'm tired of being perceived as a "bitch" in this relationship… We're worlds apart re: financial issues. I am not very hopeful, but I am grateful for all of your assistance and especially for your support.

When I moved out, Jim realized for the first time that our marriage was under siege. He relented and wrote the following apologetic letter.

I have a great deal of respect and admiration for you, Lembi and I do know how difficult I can be to live with at times… I promise to be a little more understanding when you are hiding under your stoic mask but suffering deeply. For this, I am very, very sorry.

Obviously, your health and happiness are paramount, not only to you, but also to me. I do not want to cause any undue stress. I thought that our relationship, under the circumstances, considering the health and financial issues that we have had and continue to face – to be a very solid one. Have I perceived wrongly? Surely after all that we have gone through, we are able to deal with the issues at hand. You are far too important to me for anything to interfere. Be it resolved I am prepared to abide with whatever agreements, pertaining to financial matters (including credit cards, future income et al) that we have previously entered into, either verbally or written. I love you and need you at home beside me.

With a great deal of love and affection – always, Jim

In less than a week, we were in a lawyer's office transferring the deed of the house to my name. While we were there, I also had Jim sign forms granting me Power of Attorney for Property and Power of Attorney for Personal Care. I was aware that Jim only agreed to sign the legally binding documents because he knew that he could cancel them at any time. At least the house was safe.

Jim's moods continued their unpredictable course. While Epival may have mitigated against a resurgence of manic symptoms, the mood stabilizer was not having an impact as far as quelling some of the crippling anxiety Jim was experiencing on an ongoing basis. As a last resort, Dr. Margetts prescribed Ativan (lorazepam) to take at night. The anti-anxiety drug is a benzodiazepine medication in the same family as Valium and Librium, but far more potent. For some time, Ativan was also an effective sleep aide. As winter began to set in, however, Jim was becoming anxious again. Once again, we were running out of options. As long as the drug enabled Jim to sleep through the night, we had no choice but to weather the storm.

David and Goliath

Jim always believed that Prudential would eventually pay his disability benefits. Just the same, he knew that taking on the "Rock of Gibraltar," the largest insurance company in North America, would be a formidable task.

When Jim refused to settle, Prudential requested an independent medical evaluation, requiring him to travel to Toronto for an appointment with a psychiatrist selected by the insurer. I insisted that Prudential also cover all expenses for Jonathan to accompany his father since he was not well enough to travel on his own. As it turned out, the trip was very stressful for Jim, who described his meeting with Dr. Alfred Margulies as an "interrogation." Notwithstanding his position as a witness for Prudential, Dr. Margulies presented an honest evaluation of Jim's condition, noting the following in his report to the insurer:

Bipolar illness, in contrast to earlier understanding, is now believed to result, at times, in some, ongoing symptomology that may persist following a remission of the acute or depressive episode and may leave the individual with a greater or lesser degree of dysfunction... At this point, there would appear to be little doubt but that Mr. Buchanan is vocationally disabled and he runs a high risk that he may remain as such for an indeterminate period of time.

The trial was set for three days, starting Monday morning, on February 13, 1995. Tensions were already building up during breakfast in the crowded restaurant at the Holiday Inn where all parties involved with the case appeared to be staying. Harold Beaudry, a Queen's Counsel and senior trial lawyer from Sudbury and Mitchell Marcus, representing Prudential were discussing Jim's case with one of their witnesses at a nearby table. While we couldn't make out the details of their conversation, their presence had an unnerving effect on both of us. Jim's hands were shaking so badly that he could barely drink his coffee. My stomach was tied in knots.

Judge M. DiSalle laid down the ground rules for his court right from the beginning, with the following caveat: "Proceed carefully. We're dealing with mental illness." Even so, it was evident that Prudential's legal team got off on the wrong foot with Judge DiSalle. They were very professional, smooth, and even tried to charm me when I was on the witness stand. They were also arrogant and disrespectful on several occasions, and it was clear that Judge DiSalle was not amused.

The key witnesses for Jim were his personal physician, Dr. Margetts as well as Dr. Cooke, who would be able to provide detailed testimony regarding Jim's mental state covering the period from November 1992 to the present. Their testimony would be countered by Dr. Margulies, who had only seen Jim once. They all faced the same dilemma: was it possible that Jim's mental state had miraculously improved to the degree that he could carry out all his responsibilities within six months of his hospitalization in December 1990?

Jim agreed to testify on his own behalf. He was not about to be intimidated when Prudential's lawyers cross examined him. Despite the effects of a severe mental illness on his overall well-being, Jim was an experienced communicator, and they were no match for him. Jim had already won his case when appealing his involuntary status at Toronto General Hospital in December 1990. When Mr. Beaudry realized that he wasn't scoring any points for Prudential, he quickly dismissed Jim after a few questions.

Jim's boss for the past ten years, Richard (Dick) Diotte, was also a key witness for Prudential. There was considerable time spent on the details of Jim's job description during the difficult months when two of the company's three mines in Elliot Lake began to shut down. Mr. Diotte confirmed that Jim, in addition to his normal responsibilities, handled all media inquiries as well as the "hotline" set up in his office for general inquiries from the community. He testified that "Jim just wasn't himself" when invited to come to the office for a meeting in May 1991, noting that "he seemed to be withdrawn and it was difficult to communicate with him."

The following morning over breakfast, Mr. Kearns informed us that Prudential was offering Jim a settlement of $150,000 plus $20,000 to cover his legal expenses. Our immediate concern was tax implications for such a lump sum payment and therefore, it was not as attractive as it might have appeared. Mr. Kearns probably suspected that there was no chance of being fully compensated for his services if he lost the case. Nonetheless, he was confident of a win and recommended that we go back to court.

In a last-ditch effort, Mr. Marcus attempted to discredit my testimony by introducing the Supreme Court of Canada ruling of *Regina v. Abbey 1982*. While handing out photocopies of the case, Mr. Marcus cautioned the judge about giving too much weight to my observations of Jim's mental state. However, there was no comparison between the two legal battles. The accused, Robert Mark Abbey, was characterized as a "hypomaniac" dealing in cocaine. His mother's testimony, when describing her son's mental state to his psychiatrist,

138

was ruled as hearsay evidence since she never appeared in court to substantiate her account. My testimony, on the other hand, was given in court, under oath, and accepted by Judge DiSalle as "straightforward" and "truthful."

In his closing arguments, Mr. Marcus also attempted to invalidate Jim's testimony, citing that his own doctor testified that he couldn't rely on Jim for an accurate description of his symptoms. As if that mattered, since Jim's tendency to minimize the severity of his symptoms should have been advantageous to Prudential's case. Also, Mr. Marcus made a specific reference to the numerous hardships that we had endured in recent years, suggesting that Judge DiSalle should be careful not to let his sympathies get in the way of his decision.

Just in case such a subtle warning wasn't direct enough, Mr. Marcus continued to elaborate why Judge DiSalle should dismiss Jim's claim. Citing Dr. Cooke's testimony, he reminded the judge that one per cent of the population was diagnosed with manic-depressive illness; a favourable decision for Jim would be detrimental to insurers and employers since it would "open the flood gates to new cases." Judge DiSalle took offense and said so. "Are you trying to scare me?" he asked in disbelief.

Two long agonizing months passed before we received Judge DiSalle's decision:

The evidence of Dr. Cooke, Mrs. Buchanan, Mr. Buchanan and Mr. Diotte, all of which I accept, proves on a balance of probabilities that the plaintiff has been continuously totally disabled from his episode in 1990-1991 to the present.

The victory lifted Jim's spirits.

We managed to pay off all our debts except for the mortgage on the house. I wrote a note with a cheque to Jim's parents thanking them again for their unwavering support. For the time being, the financial stressors that threatened to create a rift in our relationship had disappeared.

As far as Jim was concerned, there was every reason to celebrate. And so we did, as soon as I was able to arrange some vacation time. We toured the American Southwest and sampled some of the finest cuisine in each state. On our way home, we spent a weekend at the historic Grand Hotel on Mackinac Island in Northern Michigan, behaving like newlyweds with a renewed commitment to each other. Even during the darkest days of our marriage, I never doubted Jim's love for me. There were still moments of tenderness, and the same sensual desire, when lying in bed beside him, and he would take my hand, and squeeze it ever so gently.

Christmas cruise

Jim loved to surprise me.

On December 1, our 22nd wedding anniversary, he had taped a picture of a cruise ship inside his card with the details of a Christmas holiday in the Caribbean with both children. Jim had been secretly planning the trip for months and everyone knew about the upcoming cruise, except me. Jim also had the foresight to discuss his plans with my business partner. Her approval was critical since I was already scheduled to work the week between Christmas and New Year's.

As much as I worried about Jim's extravagant spending, I needed to spend time with Jonathan and Larissa. They had been away at boarding school since they were 12 years old, and now both were attending university. An uninterrupted week with them was a luxury I was prepared to accept without complaint.

Most importantly, Jim was well, and we had a fabulous time. We participated as a family in many of the events on board ship, just losing by a point in the Trivial Pursuit contest. And teaming up with others in shuffleboard tournaments. Nothing, however, was more relaxing than the four of us lying on our deck chairs beside the pool sipping piña coladas. There was none of the tension between Jonathan and his father that had threatened to drive a wedge in their relationship during the summer when he was home from university.

All of us also loved getting dressed up for the evening dinners. On Christmas day, a very nice California Chardonnay was brought to our table with the compliments of the President and CEO of the Holland America Line.

"President?" I asked Jim. "How do we rate?"

Jim just smiled. Clearly, he was enjoying the moment. Later he sheepishly confessed, explaining that he had written the President advising him that I had terminal cancer (which was true) and it may be my last Christmas with my family (which was also true). No wonder we were given free upgrades, from the two purchased cabins on the lower E level to more spacious cabins on the C level. We were also provided with a quiet corner table for dinner throughout the cruise.

So, I wasn't surprised when we were also invited to a small private reception hosted by the ship's captain. It was a select group, a few travel agents and passengers who had been on at least ten prior cruises with Holland America. I felt embarrassed. Was the captain aware of my "deteriorating" health condition? Is that why he was so attentive? Was it wrong to feel special? I grew up in a working-class environment and it was easy to be seduced by wealth and status when we had neither. However, Jim grew up in a privileged environment and had plenty of chutzpah to open many doors for us. When we were back home, Jim sent the President a thank you note.

I couldn't remember being as happy as I was, cruising the Caribbean Sea and visiting sun-soaked islands. We were the picture-perfect family in the photos taken during our cruise that I still treasure.

There were also moments when we faced the awful realization that Jim may never fully recover from the ravages of a disease that can cause the same progressive brain damage seen in neurodegenerative diseases like Alzheimer's and Parkinson's. One night, we went to the library with a set of dominoes that I had given Jim as a gift. Instead of numbers, each of the 28 wooden pieces were beautifully painted with colourful stick drawings taken from Miro's avant-garde art. Larissa teamed up with Jim while Jonathan and I would challenge them. Jim was having a terrible time. Although dominoes is a simple game that young children play, he found the drawings confusing and couldn't remember the rules.

I was shocked and disheartened at Jim's loss of cognitive function, no doubt, eroding slowly with each manic/depressive episode. It was the first time I realized that Jim no longer had the same capacity to process new information. When we got home, I reviewed the assessment report after two days of intensive testing at The Clarke in January 1993 to determine his employment potential. The report noted that Jim had problems with concentration and "appeared to have some difficulty with the instructions with the simpler, more common tasks." His verbal skills were in the "high average" range but he had considerable difficulty with many of the reasoning tests.

Was it any wonder that the Ontario Ministry of Community and Social Services rejected Jim's application for vocational rehabilitation services? In addition to the dismal test results, Jim was advised that he was "at high risk for a subsequent manic or depressive episode relapse."

And yet, Jim didn't seem to have any difficulty planning and making all the reservations for cross border trips without the aid of a travel agent, or our Christmas cruise that year, or subsequent years, for that matter. He was a stickler for details and always prepared a well-organized binder that contained all the reservations and maps of our destinations. Nothing was ever left to chance.

Chapter Seven – Betrayal

Manic money meltdown

If I was really smart, I would have bailed out long ago. But I was still crazy in love with someone who, I believed, also loved me just as much. Granted, there were several missteps along the way, leaving me confused and angry. The pain was all the more intense, when it was obvious that Jim didn't care about my emotional distress.

As much as I tried to distance myself from Jim's irresponsible and reckless spending habits, I found myself implicated nonetheless, as he so aptly noted in an email:

It is still rather mystifying that a bright woman like yourself can live a lifestyle that obviously costs more than the family budget (can afford). Was this simply a matter of "ignorance is bliss?"

Jim's brother John was quite blunt in his assessment of my predicament:

I fail to understand how you can allow yourself to be controlled by Jim to the extent that it seems you have… I know that you can't be a babysitter all of the time, but it appears that Jim and the concept of economic responsibility have yet to be introduced to each other… But then, what do I know?

What do I know? Not much it seems.

And yet, both were telling me that I should have known better. Like it or not, I would be branded as an enabler, or worse, an accomplice, contributing to Jim's financial crises. I had no one to blame but myself. It's complicated, like everything else in our lives. Even now, it is impossible to understand the depths of deception that threatened our marriage all over again.

The complexity of bipolar disorder cannot be overstated. As difficult as it is to explain the impact of this mysterious brain disease on the decision-making process of an individual, it is far more difficult to excuse when we're talking about money.

The banking industry has had its own love affair with Jim for many years and still does. It never seemed to matter if Jim was gainfully employed or not. Whenever he requested a credit card, it materialized, as if by magic, in the mail, and always in a plain envelope.

No sooner had we unpacked our bags from our Christmas cruise when Jim informed me that we were going to California for a week at the end of February. He was eager to share the good news, especially since he had managed to secure hard-to-get tickets for the annual Masters of Food & Wine event held at the Highlands Inn in Carmel.

I was stunned. Once again, I had not been consulted. Apparently, it never occurred to Jim that I might not want to go. After all, the last snow fall in Elliot Lake was almost knee-deep. Sub-zero night-time temperatures required us to plug in our vehicles to an electrical supply if we wanted to go anywhere in the morning. On the other hand, flowers were already in bloom in Carmel. Was there really any reason to say, no? I couldn't think of it, so I happily packed our bags with appropriate evening wear and Jim rented a tux for the Grand Finale Dinner.

Our elegant and spacious spa suite was perched high up on the hill, with a breath-taking view of the craggy coastline of the Pacific Ocean. A wood-burning fireplace was the centrepiece of the living area, and a family-sized Jacuzzi dominated the opposite corner of the suite. I had never experienced such luxury in a so-called "rustic" setting that must have cost a fortune. I was afraid to ask, so I didn't. After all, Jim had received a substantial cheque from Prudential. Rather than obsessing about the cost, I unpacked and quickly dressed for the evening reception.

Let's be honest. I enjoy good food and fine wines as much as Jim. And the culinary excitement of the event was evident with dozens of chefs showcasing dazzling new taste sensations along with some of the best wines from local vineyards. Jim couldn't be happier, mingling with an international crowd of food and wine connoisseurs.

I was shamelessly caught up as well, gloating over the most extraordinary spread of haute cuisine on this side of paradise.

We socialized with a most congenial group of foodies and our conversations were dominated by sumptuous courses, each paired with a spectacular wine. All lunches and dinners were "intimate affairs" with table settings for 160 guests at round tables of eight who were quite prepared to swoon over roasted lobster prepared with morel mushrooms and paired with a German Riesling.

There was a certain camaraderie as we banded together, when served a not so brilliant California Pinot Noir with a distinct barnyard nose that was swiftly rejected by our table. "A real dud!" we echoed as a waiter hastily removed the offensive bottle, replacing it with another for our enjoyment, as we feasted on Colorado loin of lamb with pancetta and foie gras.

In addition to the luncheons and dinners, I signed up for cooking demonstrations. At 86, Julia Child was as witty as ever, preparing pan roasted duckling and serving it with pearl onions and sliced polenta that she found at a Boston market. "It's really very good," she said, not at all apologetic, when referring to Rosa's ready-made packaged polenta imported from Canada. When someone asked her about low-fat sour cream, she turned up her nose and suggested that the real deal was much better. Jacques Pepin, another popular chef and television personality taught us the basics of how to make an unforgettable apple tarte tatin.

Our week in California was way over the top from a personal financial perspective. But then, I wasn't picking up the tab. I was just happy to see that Jim was also enjoying himself. We both agreed that life was too short not to take advantage of pleasurable, even indulgent experiences, whenever possible. We were both painfully conscious of our close calls with our physical and mental health with no guarantees of our future well-being.

And so, Jim and I would escape the frigid temperatures of Canadian winters, returning to California every February for a number of years.

Jim also managed to find more affordable accommodations at the Green Lantern Inn, a charming B & B in Carmel that had been an artist's colony in the 1920s. A most prudent decision, a few years later, considering the hedonistic extravagance of the James House Rarities Wine Dinner.

Jim was "lucky enough" to have his name drawn for the opportunity to purchase two tickets for the lavish seven-course meal paired with some of the finest vintages in the world. In his "Gourmet's Paradise" column in the British publication *Decanter*, food and wine critic, Father Francis Bown confessed that he had missed out on the "grandest dinner of the week" as "two dozen lotus-eaters sat down to a repast accompanied by such wines that dreams are made of..." We had met Father Bown earlier that day, during lunch, when he confided that his magazine wasn't prepared to shell out $2,000 per person for a once in a lifetime experience. Of course, Jim had never intended to disclose the cost since he knew I would strenuously object to such an exorbitant price tag for dinner for just the two of us.

As we waited for our shuttle bus to take us to the James House, I was feeling particularly dowdy, shivering in my London Fog trench coat among beautifully dressed women, some with mink jackets to ward off the chill. Now owned by Brad Pitt, the historic mansion, built on a cliff with the roar of the surf below us, was the perfect location for such an indulgent meal. Once inside, I wasted no time checking my coat. And as Father Bown so aptly wrote in his column: "With such miracles of gastronomy on show, there was nothing to do but enjoy."

I was caught up in an impossible situation. In many ways, I was grateful that Jim took on the responsibility of planning our trips, booking our flights, car rentals and accommodations. He always spent considerable time online on research, trying to get the best deals to stretch our travel dollar. However, he was also making reservations at innovative new restaurants featured in *Gourmet* magazine, which we really couldn't afford. I wrote about my frustrations in my journal, feeling guilty when ordering from some of the pricier menus:

146

I am trapped. I have no choice… My head spins, after paying tax, tip and converting the bill into Canadian dollars. I am not even sure if I am enjoying myself – I feel somewhat responsible for Jim's extravagances. And yet, I have no control over his behaviour. The few times, when I want something, I'm almost afraid to ask. Thank goodness we didn't go to San Diego. I would have been completely worn out from that trip. When Jim mentioned that the only reason to drive down the coast was to dine at the famous Hotel del Coronado, I objected, advising him that it would take us all day just to drive there.

I was relieved when we headed north, back to San Francisco for the last few days of our California holiday and settled in at Albion House, a modest B & B near the Civic Center. Once again, the pace was daunting with so many extraordinary meals and blockbuster wines. I had trouble keeping up with Jim and by the end of each evening, I was exhausted. Not Jim. One night, he ordered a second brandy snifter of Cognac as well as a cigar. I knew better than to say anything right then and there. Once we arrived back at our room, I unleashed my frustration in an angry tirade. And then I apologized for lashing out at him.

Why would I apologize? It should have been obvious that Jim wasn't well. While he may have seemed "normal" to others, I believe that he was experiencing unpredictable shifts in mood, mixed states, alternating between manic and depressive symptoms. Sometimes, I wondered if both manic and depressed states could be present simultaneously.

Buying six pairs of an expensive brand of wool knee-high socks at Macy's was one thing. Crossing the street to Neiman Marcus and spending $86 for a bottle of wine in the specialty shop was another matter, and a prime example of how Jim was unstoppable. I was right there, reminding him that we were already over our limit as far as the number of bottles we were taking back home with us. Jim didn't care. He exercised little or no restraint over impulsive purchases. The wine was "an essential purchase from an important vintner" and that was all that mattered.

There was absolutely nothing I could have said, or threatened, to prevent Jim's excessive spending sprees. The manic mind has no insight into practical matters such as affordability. Naturally, I could not abandon him when he was in an unstable state. Not when we were thousands of miles away from home.

That night, after dinner at the Ritz Carleton Hotel, I suggested to Jim he had too much to drink to drive back to the B & B. Instead of handing over the car keys, he snarled at me: "Are you the angel of God?" I was afraid to say anything else and prayed that we would get back safely to our lodgings.

The following morning, while I was packing our bags, Jim went to pick up our rental car which was parked on the next block. He came back 20 minutes later, saying he couldn't remember where he had left the car. That was hardly surprising, considering his inebriated state the previous evening. Panic stricken, I grabbed the keys from his hand, found our car and was back at our lodgings in five minutes flat.

As we were leaving the Albion House for the airport, Jim was complaining about the weight of our suitcases. What did he expect? I had already packed six bottles of wine into two suitcases including the prized magnum of Heitz Cellars Cabernet Sauvignon we had received from friends. In a last-ditch effort, Jim decided to check out another store for a rare bottle of 1961 French Armagnac; thankfully it wasn't available.

I wasn't the only one frustrated over Jim's freewheeling spending habits. His father certainly expected that his lectures over the years would have some influence over his son's ability to deal with finances in a more responsible manner. The science, however, tells a different story, that the manic mind is unlike the workings of the normal brain with its checks and balances. According to the Diagnostic and Statistical Manual of Mental Disorders (5th ed.), one of the symptoms of mania is "excessive involvement in pleasurable activities with high potential for painful consequence (e.g., engaging in unrestrained buying sprees, sexual indiscretions, or foolish business investments)."

There is plenty of advice online on how to limit the damage of uncontrolled manic spending sprees. While recommendations by well-meaning, so-called experts may look good in print, they are not always realistic, certainly not, for someone like Jim. Surely, he is not alone. I thought I had taken all the right steps early in our relationship. Even so, it has never been easy to follow hard and fast rules, or set specific boundaries, if not for Jim, but for myself.

Nor is there is a shortage of memoirs where authors diagnosed with bipolar disorder describe their manic spending sprees. In *An Unquiet Mind*, Kay Redfield Jamison, an American psychologist affiliated with the Johns Hopkins University School of Medicine, provides an insight into how easy it is to spend "a lot of money you don't have."

When I am high, I couldn't worry about money if I tried. So I don't. The money will come from somewhere; I am entitled; God will provide... What with credit cards and bank accounts (with generous credit limits), there is little beyond reach... mania is not a luxury one can easily afford.

How is it possible to draw the line when the manic mind knows no bounds?

A life in limbo

In May 1996, both Larissa and Jonathan had just come home from university and were excited about celebrating my 50th birthday at the end of the month, a truly remarkable milestone for me. We decided we could cram at least 25 friends for a buffet dinner in our home. Predictably, Jim was obsessing over the choice of wines to serve with the meal.

We had every reason to celebrate. My life had been in limbo for so many years, worrying about the results of annual CT scans as well as continuing to take powerful hormonal medications to prevent further tumour growth. Jim said it best one day: "Maybe God doesn't want you." That may be true, but perhaps he didn't realize that God was aware Jim needed someone to look after him.

Of course, Jim would vehemently deny that he needed a caregiver. Whatever he might want others to believe, all was not well. Jim was becoming increasingly irritable and argumentative. I could not let go of the painful realization that his impulsive hurtful behaviour in front of his children, was symptomatic of a disease that he had little, if any control over. Still, I was deeply wounded by his insensitive outbursts. When I asked Jim to be more civil, at least towards Jonathan and Larissa, he told me to "fuck off." Then he added, for good measure, "You can't hospitalize me." The message was loud and clear. Jim was off the rails again.

Naturally, he was right. His symptoms were not severe enough to lock him up since he was not exhibiting signs that he might be a danger to himself or others. I spent the night on the couch and Jim retaliated by locking me out of the bedroom. He apologized the following day when I came home from work. "There's a truce between the two of us," I noted in my journal, with some skepticism, adding, "We'll see how long it lasts."

Days prior to my birthday, Jim and Larissa went shopping for a new barbecue, not as a gift for me, but for him. When Jim was experiencing manic symptoms, everything was about him. Larissa was shocked at the $999 price tag for the Napoleon gas grill and suggested to her father that he could save $300 by purchasing a smaller model by the same manufacturer. Jim wasn't listening. If he wanted something, no one could stand in his way. Not me, and certainly not his daughter. Jim had to have the best in the showroom and money was no object. Or so it seemed.

My 50th birthday celebration was a "tremendous success" according to my journal entry. Everyone, it seemed, had a wonderful time, except for Jim. He was restless, getting up from the table more than once and shuffling around the room, eventually disappearing without a word into the bedroom. When Larissa brought out the cake, there were plenty of toasts and well wishes from our friends. They, along with my extraordinary children, refused to let Jim's unpredictable and bizarre behaviour ruin an unforgettable day, reminding me how much I was loved. Jonathan and Larissa also loved their father, despite his disagreeable behaviour at times. On the other hand, Jim could be very generous, taking them twice to California during March break when I was unable to get away. One year, while staying at a hotel in San Francisco, he surprised them with a 5:00 am wake-up call to drive to Napa Valley for a hot-air balloon ride. Jim also stood in line for hours to pick up $10 front row tickets for the new musical *Rent* when it opened in Toronto in 1997. On a whim, he picked up tickets for them to attend a U2 concert when the Irish rock band was performing in the city. On the flip side, Jim could be very demanding, insisting on appropriate table manners, even at home, and excellent grades at school. There was always a sense of helplessness on my part when Jim was unduly harsh with the kids.

In her English composition exam, while in high school, Larissa wrote the following essay, with the understanding that her father's illness was impossible to define or understand:

People are not always who they seem to be on the outside, but they all know how to love. My father is no exception; he tries his best in life. He doesn't always succeed, and there are many factors that keep him from reaching his destination... A wall has been erected between him and everyone else. One tries to scale it and look on the other side, but no one can ever succeed... believe me, I have tried... It's difficult for everyone in the family... The illness is not a noticeable feature, but it's always in my mind...

As I sit here writing down thoughts of my life with my father, tension grows inside of me. I'm left confused, wondering when his next episode will be, and how I will be affected... My mother asks me to be a little more sensitive with him at times, but I can't let his illness drag me down. Everything I say to my father is not always going to be positive... I don't want to upset him, but I don't want to have a lot of things build up inside me.

I wasn't nearly as understanding.

Our relationship remained strained that summer. While cleaning under the bed one day, I came across statements from two credit card companies charged right up to their limits. How could Jim be in debt when he was receiving a decent monthly disability income? When I expressed my dismay, Jim didn't care. As usual, he refused to take any responsibility for his actions. As far as he was concerned, I was the only one with a problem.

Sometimes, I wondered if I was going mad. Otherwise, how could I put up with a husband who blamed me whenever money was tight. Was I truly at fault? After all, he reminded me time and time again, if I wasn't paying for Jonathan and Larissa's tuition at university as well as their room and board, we wouldn't be struggling financially. I knew deep down inside that I was treading on dangerous ground whenever I started to give Jim the benefit of doubt. Under normal circumstances, he would be right. There was no reason why our children couldn't apply for student loans and pay their own way. That would greatly ease our financial burden and perhaps, allow us to set some savings aside for retirement. But the reality was plain and simple: if I wasn't supporting Jonathan and Larissa, Jim would have "sucked up" my earnings one way or the other.

At the end of August, Jim drove Jonathan and Larissa back to Toronto. I was grateful that both of them had been home for the summer. If I accomplished anything worth bragging about, it was keeping the family together, despite a difficult summer that left me anxious about our future. Now that the kids had left for school, I was alone and feeling sorry for myself, hiding my private pain in a journal entry.

Does anyone know how much it hurts when you're sobbing inside and no one is listening? I just can't cry about anything anymore. Not for several years. There doesn't seem anything worth crying about when no one is listening. Certainly not Jim. He can be so terribly cruel. And what's worse, he doesn't care.

That was then.

My next journal notation was a week later when Jim returned from Toronto. His mood had improved considerably. He was less irritable and confrontational, no longer arguing about trivial matters. Jim was also becoming more active in the community, volunteering his services on various mental health committees. Most importantly, he was more attentive to my needs, trying to ease some of the pressures at home while I was struggling to keep ELMAR Company afloat.

Our love had endured another dark chapter. The romance was rekindled. Our relationship was as good as it ever was, and we were lovers once more. Still, the possibility of a relapse was always a concern as my journal entry at the end of September noted the insecurity I was living with:

Jim is in a rare mood… more pleasant and lively than he has been in years. I'm not used to so much activity. But we have been there before – when suddenly everything is terrific for awhile and then he's in another stratosphere. How high can he go this time? Or am I just needlessly worrying. We shall see…

As it turned out, there was no reason to worry. Jim was well. I was delighted when he booked another Christmas cruise in the Caribbean for our family. Not surprisingly, both Jonathan and Larissa were thrilled as well. We had a wonderful week at sea, and we were all in agreement that it was another "perfect" holiday.

25 years of marital bliss

We moved back to Toronto in August 1997. Despite efforts to secure new markets for our products when the local mining industry collapsed, I wasn't confident that ELMAR Company could survive the economic downturn of our town. I cashed in my interest in the once profitable manufacturing business and we put up our house for sale. Jim went on a reconnaissance trip hoping to find a suitable rental apartment in his old neighbourhood. He would have preferred to look at condominiums, since he believed that renting was synonymous with throwing money down the drain. That may be true for some people, but not for us. I was afraid, if Jim ever had to declare bankruptcy, that we might lose our home. As far as Jim was concerned, I was over-reacting. After all, wasn't he well? Just the same, I was relieved when Jim found a lovely three-bedroom apartment, a few blocks north of Casa Loma with a stunning view of the CN Tower and Lake Ontario from our bedroom.

With some money in the bank from the sale of the house after paying off the mortgage, I suggested that we consider a Mediterranean cruise. Jim didn't need any convincing and found an exciting ten-day itinerary of the Greek isles, from Istanbul to Athens, including several days in Israel. He also opted for a surprisingly modest upgrade to business class for our flights. The upgrade to the owners' suite on the *Aegean I* was another matter though Jim assured me that it was a very good deal.

We had no sooner boarded an Air Alitalia flight when Jim started to make a fuss. In all fairness to him, the seating plan was unconventional, and we were separated by an aisle with Jim in a single seat beside the window. He called the flight attendant over and insisted that she seat us together. Jim had already had a few drinks while we were waiting in the lounge and was in a confrontational mood. Regrettably, with a full cabin, there were no other options. Jim didn't care and demanded to know the name of the president of the airline. The flight attendant was not about to put up with Jim's rude behaviour. She leaned over him and said, very sternly, "It's a long flight to Rome and we may as well get along. Otherwise, you will be escorted off the plane when we stop in Montreal." I couldn't believe what I was hearing. She was threatening to kick Jim off the plane if he didn't calm down. I was terrified that Jim would jeopardize our vacation with his impulsive angry outbursts.

Cocktails were served as soon as we were airborne; thankfully Jim had already drifted off and was sound asleep. "Is he always like that?" the flight attendant asked me. She must have sensed that I felt terribly embarrassed because I didn't respond. "I would have kicked him out long ago," she whispered in my ear.

I had always worried about Jim's alcohol intake in airport lounges with an open bar. It was the same story at social functions. I had never been successful asking him to limit his drinking when it was obvious that he had already had more than he should. When confronting Jim about abusing alcohol, he could become obnoxious, mean, nasty and, sometimes, threatening. So, it was hardly surprising that he lashed out at me, when we were back in New York, a few months later celebrating our wedding anniversary.

Jim had planned the trip as a surprise. At the time, I was thrilled when Jim finally let the cat out of the bag. Who wouldn't be? I loved New York during the Christmas season. And yet, even before we left town, I woke up in a cold sweat one night, worrying about the cost. The Canadian dollar was at an all-time low, so anything "expensive" would be translated immediately into "extravagant" on Jim's credit card bill.

There was no turning back. The hotel was already booked and paid for. Lunch and dinner reservations at some of the city's best restaurants had been made months ago. Jim had also purchased tickets for two Broadway shows.

Prior to the matinee performance of *Triumph of Love,* we sat down for drinks at the bar at Sardi's. The iconic celebrity watering hole had been catering to the Broadway crowd for 75 years, with caricatures of stars lining the walls. The waiter took our orders: a Perrier for me and a double Scotch for Jim. I was afraid to say anything since he was in unusually good spirits after an excellent lunch and a fine bottle of wine. The musical was a fantasy, where love triumphed over incredible odds, much like our own relationship.

On our last night in New York, Jim chose the Rainbow Room at the top of Rockefeller Center for a nightcap. The elegant restaurant was one of the most romantic spots in New York for dining and dancing. There was no denying that Jim had a gift for making me feel very special, as we lingered over a bottle of wine, when he reached across the table, taking my hand gently, and saying, "I love you."

However, it was a different story on the following day. After lunch with one of Jim's friends, we were in a cab on our way to the airport, when the "love of my life" suddenly turned on me. I can't recall our conversation, but I must have crossed the line. Jim was furious. His eyes were cold and hard as he warned me: "Stop it, or I'll belt you across the face."

I was stunned. It was déjà vu in the very worst sense. Jim had reacted the same way, it seemed so long ago but not forgotten, in February 1973. We were in a cab crossing Central Park on our way home from a very late dinner at the Ginger Man. Back then, Jim carried out his threat. Afraid that he might do so again, I retreated to the corner of my seat and kept quiet for the remainder of the cab ride. I felt ashamed, as if it was somehow my fault. Otherwise, how could a generous, loving husband suddenly turn on his wife in such a terrifying manner?

Earlier in the day, I met Jim and his friend for lunch at Lutèce, one of the city's finest French restaurants, with one of the best wine cellars on the continent. It was quite evident that they had already been drinking, and I worried that Jim might become obnoxious, and spoil our lunch. Perhaps Jim was trying to impress his friend, not only with his choice of restaurant, but also his vast knowledge of wines. As we raised our glasses, I was stunned when Jim casually mentioned the $200 price tag for the vintage Burgundy accompanying our meal.

Alas, Lutèce had been downgraded by *The New York Times* since we were there more than ten years ago, from four to three stars. So, it was hardly surprising that there were a few empty tables scattered about the dining room. As it was, the lamb with the black trumpet mushrooms, even the French onion soup, were disappointing. Or maybe, I was just too anxious to enjoy my meal, feeling guilty because the tab would easily exceed our monthly grocery tab.

Jim was polite when asking the waiter for the bill, though his speech was pressured, a common indicator of a significant shift in mood. There was every reason to be concerned on more than one front.

Especially, when a very apologetic waiter informed Jim that his credit card had been declined. I can't remember feeling so embarrassed in front of others, as if I was somehow responsible for the lack of funds to cover the lunch tab. I had no choice but to reach for my purse to pay for our meal. Jim was quicker, opening up his wallet again, pulling out another credit card and, without a word, handing it to waiter. I dreaded the day when the house of cards would collapse around him.

I tried not to let Jim's crass behaviour in the cab on the way to the airport detract from the wonderful moments we had shared that week. When Jim finally sobered up, he apologized without a hint of remorse. Back home, he added the following note in my journal: "I have nothing to explain. A bit too much alcohol might alter normal responses – hardly anything to worry about."

But I did worry.

The very concept of being impaired was foreign to Jim. Nor did he believe that he had a problem with alcohol dependency. He didn't understand how easily an extra glass of wine could lead to another and another and inevitably to major shifts in his mood, from being a caring loving husband to an angry hostile stranger. I was also afraid that Jim might become violent if he felt threatened in any way. I had to be careful not be confrontational in public, even if it meant tolerating a certain degree of psychological abuse. Fortunately, these encounters were rare, mostly forgotten and always forgiven.

As much as I was surprised when Jim had managed to arrange the trip to New York in secret, I was caught completely off guard a year later, with a call from the Reverend Canon Milton Barry of Grace Church on-the-Hill. He explained that there were still a few details that needed to be finalized regarding the ceremony for the renewal of our vows on our 25th wedding anniversary. Apparently, Jim had already arranged for an organist to play during the service and a pianist for the reception. All I had to do was approve the program and send out the invitations.

I didn't know whether to laugh or cry. I certainly wasn't prepared to ask Jim how much such an elaborate service followed by a reception in the church library was going to cost. I already knew that money was no object when Jim was determined to follow through with his plans.

As expected, I could count on his organizational skills, ensuring a wonderful celebration in every way for our family and friends who were unable to attend our wedding in New York. Every detail was perfect, from the organ selections of Henry Purcell's "Trumpet Tune," as we walked down the centre aisle holding hands, and to the joyful strains of Charles Widor's "Toccata" from Symphony V, at the end of the service. Our friend Ann chose the traditional reading of Corinthians 13: 4-8 for weddings from *The Living Bible*:

Love is ever patient and kind, never jealous or envious, boastful or proud, never haughty or selfish or rude. Love does not demand its own way. It is not irritable or touchy. It does not hold grudges and will hardly even notice when others do it wrong. It is never glad about injustice but rejoices whenever truth wins out. If you love someone, you will be loyal to him no matter what the cost. You will always believe in him, always expect the best of him and always stand your ground in defending him.

During the reception, the pianist entertained us with some of our favourite selections from various Broadway shows, including Stephen Sondheim's "Send in the Clowns" from *A Little Night Music*. There was every reason to be joyful as we celebrated "25 years of marital bliss" with the following words on the back cover of our program:

Over the years,
it is love that sustains us.
The love of God.
The love of family.
And, just as important,
the love of friends.

Jim and I were two people who truly loved each other, despite our struggles and shortcomings. And yet, our love was only as strong as the love of our family and friends who stood by us, never judging and always supportive. We would need to be able to count on them again and again.

Limited legal liability

While Jim spent his time plotting and planning our next trips, I left him alone. I was busy with contracts with his former employer, Rio Algom, developing communications strategies and materials related to the mine closures. The company's reclamation efforts included returning its properties back to nature along with the protection of the extensive Serpent River Watershed that emptied into Lake Huron.

I was also looking for a full-time communications position with the help of an agency, but so far, I had been unsuccessful. Why was it so difficult to find a job when I wanted to work? I began to question my own sense of worth; it was painfully evident that Jim was doing the same. There was no question that we could manage on Jim's disability income and my consulting fees, if our finances were managed properly. Some nights I would lie in bed and fret about Jim's financial excesses. I was forced to concede that there was nothing to be gained by worrying about something I had no control over when so many decisions were made in secret. All too often, it was too late to reverse the damage.

While we were on a two-week cruise of the western Mediterranean in February, Jim hinted at possible bankruptcy proceedings that summer. Should I have been surprised by the news that he might be insolvent? Probably not, although Jim had always been careful to conceal the status of his financial affairs, renting a P.O. Box and keeping his bank statements in a locked drawer. Certainly, there was no indication of being broke as we dined at expensive restaurants during the three days in Lisbon before boarding our ship.

When Jim advised me that he still had another trip planned in April during the Easter holidays, I wasn't at all pleased. Days before leaving for the Outer Banks, a 300-kilometer-long string of barrier islands off the coast of North Carolina, I expressed my frustrations and fears in a journal entry:

The weekend is looming over me and I really don't want to go away. It's the first time that I have ever felt so little enthusiasm about going somewhere with Jim. Forget the fact that he is not always fair with me... I must keep him happy (in a relationship) with me at all costs. What would I do without him? Where would I be? It's a frightening thought.

I was caught in an all too familiar catch-22 scenario. Jim had already paid for our air travel, reserved a rental car and paid a non-refundable deposit for the accommodations. If I refused to join him, there was every reason to believe that Jim would not have hesitated to leave me behind.

Jim had indicated as much when he decided to see the week-long celebrated opera extravaganza of Richard Wagner's "Ring Cycle" performed in San Francisco one summer. The carefully typed message taped to the inside of a Valentine's Day card read: "You are under no perceived notion to join me, but as in everything I do... You are invited to come along." As I did not share his love affair of Wagner, I spent the days roaming the city with my camera.

I simply couldn't risk Jim travelling on his own. If he couldn't afford to pay for meals and cover other miscellaneous expenses, I still had sufficient financial reserves to pick up the tab. More than anything else, I wanted to protect the spark in our marriage that barely flickered at times.

Was it so wrong to try to restore some normalcy in our lives, to rejuvenate our relationship and rekindle the romance? Was I supposed to feel guilty for being in love with a husband who was unable to control his impulsive spending sprees, despite a crippling debt that he could no longer support? Instead, I treasured the days whenever our lives were back in sync, and we were lovers once more.

Like the shifting sands of the Outer Banks, my own reservations about the trip vanished as soon as we arrived at the Sanderling Inn Resort where Jim had booked a luxurious suite overlooking the Atlantic Ocean. A bottle of wine in a gift basket was delivered to our room and we sat on the balcony, sipping the chilled California Chardonnay. The ever-present sound of the surf rolling onto the shore soothed my anxieties. We spent the days exploring the beaches and the evenings dining by candlelight at local restaurants. Once more, the storm clouds on the horizon had receded, but not for long.

When we were back home, Jim was constantly on the phone. I was certainly curious when I overheard him checking up on flights to Hong Kong. Unknown to me, he had booked an Asian cruise and was trying to arrange our air travel. Of course, it never occurred to Jim to check with me first. I reminded him that I was taking a small business course and would not be able to go. Jim was quick to inform me that cancelling the cruise meant forfeiting his $800 deposit, as if I should be the one to feel guilty about money down the drain.

That summer, Jim was more irritable than usual, no doubt, because of the impending financial crisis when his house of cards finally came tumbling down. Jim never discussed his meeting with the bankruptcy trustee. Nor did he disclose any of the details of his debt. Perhaps it was just as well. I wondered, Should I be grateful that he kept me in the dark? Although my name did not appear on any of Jim's bank accounts, I learned later that I was expected to "kick in" some funds since it was assumed that part of the debt was due to shared expenses. That may have been true and steps could have been taken to garnish my wages if I had a full-time job. Without a secure pay cheque, I was off the hook for Jim's debt. Still, I was shocked that he could have dragged me down as well.

Did it really matter that I acknowledged feeling "terribly guilty about the money being spent" in a journal entry? However, I never considered myself as an enabler. I was powerless to reign in Jim's spending habits. Instead, I blamed the banking industry, for its irresponsible and inappropriate lending practices with unsolicited offers to satisfy the insatiable need for credit for people like Jim who were living within the constraints of a disability income. I wondered if he was simply unable to recognize the consequences of impulsive spending habits, as long as he had a full deck of credit cards from every major bank in the country.

I was just grateful that Jim was responsible about taking his medication and keeping his appointments with Dr. Cooke. Nevertheless, it was obvious that these drugs were insufficient to prevent sporadic spending sprees. Dr. Cooke was not surprised about Jim's unrepentant lack of responsible money management. In a letter dated March 8, 2001, and entered as evidence in Jim's tax court case, Dr. Cooke wrote: "Over the period that I have been involved in your care, you have shown continuous symptoms of bipolar disorder, fluctuating in severity."

Like so many bipolar partners finding themselves in compromising situations, early on I had to accept the fact that there still was no cure for manic-depressive illness. There was no choice but to keep our financial affairs separate. I paid all the expenses for the children including their school fees and contributed to our household and car expenses. But I refused to cash in my RRSPs to cover Jim's lavish spending habits. Over the years, I had managed to stash away a substantial amount from my consulting fees that morphed into $80,000. It was an important cushion considering how fractured our relationship had become. Instead of caving into Jim's insatiable need for cash, I was counting the number of subway tokens left in my wallet at the end of the month and worried whether Jim could cover the rent on the first of the following month.

A marriage under siege

"There's always the window."

Jim was lying on the bed, not bothering to look up from the afternoon newspaper.

I wasn't prepared for his curt response to my rather pathetic admission that I was depressed and didn't know what to do. I walked over to the bedroom window and looked down. A neighbour was walking her two dogs, and an older gentleman was hobbling along with a cane while clutching a bag of groceries in his other hand.

We lived on the seventh floor. Was it enough? I wondered.

If we lived on the 25th floor, there would be no question at all.

My days were as dreary as the weather, as a cloud of despair hung over me. Our marriage had been rocky for months, if not years. I had lost all interest trying to resolve our differences over finances. I had also lost hope that we could repair the damage to our relationship caused by the unrelenting emotional roller coaster of highs and lows. My heart was broken. My self-esteem had plummeted to a new low. I had lost my sense of self-respect. Nothing mattered anymore.

For more than a week, I had been trying to think of how best to approach Jim, just to let him know that I couldn't shake off the sense of hopelessness I felt about our relationship. He always seemed to be preoccupied. Either Jim didn't notice how unhappy I was, or he just didn't care.

Instead, as he suggested, I could open the window and my troubles could disappear. It was as simple as that.

I looked out of the window again. The older gentleman was gone. But our neighbour had stopped to talk to a friend while both dogs were straining at their leashes. They were anxious to move on. Would they bark if I fell at their feet?

It never occurred to me that suicide was an option, although the pain of rejection was excruciating. I had trouble coping from one day to the next. I was tired, not only of the impulsive, reckless behaviour and excessive spending, but also, the deception.

Whenever I complained about the stress he was causing in my life, Jim's response was always the same. "What about the stress you are causing me? Do you ever think of that?"

We were barely communicating with each other. If I expressed my fears that our relationship was falling apart, Jim just shrugged his shoulders and reminded me that I didn't have to stay. To make matters worse, Jim was drinking more. I was reluctant to invite anyone over to our home with the exception of family. And even then, Jim could become obnoxious and belligerent. The verbal abuse, was not only directed toward me, but also at Larissa and her friends, if any of us said something that might have offended him.

I was mindful that the impact of so many stressors affecting my overall mental health could compromise my immune system and risk a recurrence of the rare uterine cancer that was in remission. I could simply allow myself to surrender to the disease and no one would blame me. When I saw Dr. Murphy for a routine check-up in November, it was the first time I had ever lost my calm demeanour in front of her. I broke down in tears as I shared a recent journal entry with her:

Sometimes, I wish that my illness would shorten my life. I can't continue living with such anxiety… not knowing what Jim is planning or how he'll pay for the extravagant lifestyle he keeps pursuing. I can't afford to keep up with him. And I don't have the energy to fight back. I simply don't have the will to carry on anymore. There is no more joy in my life with Jim so disinterested in my well-being.

Dr. Murphy had kept me alive well beyond the five-year survival rate and was not about to lose me, not if she had any say in the matter. She also understood how easily Jim was affected by previous recurrences of illness, with him back in the hospital as well. Dr. Murphy suggested that I see a colleague of hers who was affiliated with the hospital's psychiatric department and one of the best in her field.

I was a nervous wreck for days before my appointment with Dr. Susan Abbey. My self-confidence was already shattered, and I was too embarrassed to admit that I wasn't able to say "no" to Jim, for fear of upsetting him, or worse, risk the relationship, as tenuous as it was.

What if Dr. Abbey didn't understand how difficult my life had become as much as I tried to set boundaries to prevent Jim from implicating me with his reckless spending habits? Or would she blame me for not putting my foot down, when he refused to involve me with his travel plans? Or would she chastise me, for not staying home, if necessary, to teach him a lesson?

I was the only patient in the waiting room in the late afternoon in early December, when Dr. Abbey came over and invited me into her office. The room was filled with medical texts and studies piled high on book shelves and spilling onto the floor. There was barely any space for two chairs. I was more than grateful that she could fit me into her busy schedule.

Dr. Abbey could not have been more sympathetic, while I tried to explain how discouraged I felt in a relationship that was doomed to fail after all these years. Dr. Abbey did not judge me. Instead, she was kind and understanding, as if she had heard it all before. Indeed, she marvelled that I had managed to cope as long as I had, on my own, before realizing that I had reached the breaking point. Dr. Abbey prescribed a new antidepressant, Wellbutrin (bupropion) to improve my mood. She also arranged for me to see a therapist. My sessions with Heather, a psychiatric social worker, would span two years and two months as I agonized whether my marriage was worth salvaging.

The medication dulled the pain and suppressed some of my anxiety. But I was still reeling from the fact that Jim had not consulted me before booking our flights to California in February, to attend another Masters of Food & Wine event. For good measure, he had included a weekend at the historic Mark Hopkins Hotel in San Francisco.

Jim had always been very clever as far as collecting loyalty points which covered our flights, as well as some of our accommodations. I expected that Jim was not only counting on a generous Christmas cash gift from his parents, but also on my resources to cover any shortfall since his bankruptcy proceedings had cut off his unlimited source of easy money.

It was quite evident to me that Jim was operating on another plane, living in an alternate reality. I wondered if he was in a constant hypomanic mode, while trying to justify unrestrained spending sprees. As far as Jim was concerned, he was fine, and there was no need for me to worry. Whenever I questioned his actions, Jim would remind me of his "open door policy," and that I had no obligation to stay. According to him, he signed the lease and therefore the apartment was his, definitely not mine, or ours. If I didn't "behave," Jim believed that he had the right to throw me out.

The obvious question that I wrestled with during my sessions with Heather was why I had not bailed out long ago. Truth be told, I was still madly in love with Jim. And I refused to let the symptoms of his illness ruin our relationship, as rocky as it was at times. I never doubted Jim's love for me, so I hung on.

My greatest fear was that Jim might just take off by himself, if I refused to accompany him. I had no means of judging his mental state and whether he was crazy enough to pack his own bags and head off to California on his own, again, and end up in distress, again, and requiring hospitalization, again. Although Jim was not a threat to others, I felt I had an obligation to protect Jim from himself.

When Jim was given an absolute discharge from his creditors, I was relieved to discover that filing for bankruptcy would affect his credit rating for seven years and thwart his easy access to bank cards. With the rug pulled from under his feet, there was every reason to be worried. Jim was becoming easily agitated and increasingly irritable. I wondered whether his behaviour was a response to a low-level depression and if he was self-medicating with alcohol to relieve the pain.

My journal entry described my personal trauma as I tried to cope with so much uncertainty:

Jim is drinking more and couldn't care less about my feelings...He has no idea how tortuous this life is for me. How much stress I have to live with... Sometimes I really do hate him when he says terribly nasty things...

There were none of the typical warning signs indicating that Jim fit the stereotype of an alcoholic. Essentially, Jim was a social drinker. Once, he admitted that he was an introvert and alcohol freed up his inhibitions, letting him feel more confident and relaxed in the company of others. He was right, of course, since alcohol releases serotonins and endorphins into the areas of the brain involved with pleasure and reward. But there have always been limits to Jim's tolerance for alcohol which could cause volatile shifts in his mood.

Although the association between bipolar disorder and alcohol abuse is not clearly understood, there is plenty of evidence that links both conditions to inherited traits. As far as we know, Jim's mother was never diagnosed with a specific mental illness though she experienced similar symptoms as Jim when she was hospitalized for a hysterectomy. Occasionally, she might have a glass of Dubonnet, a French aperitif during the cocktail hour and a small glass of wine with dinner. Her father, Noel Marshall, however, was a heavy drinker and rarely showed up at the offices of the family coal business. Instead, he stayed home, in the semi-darkness of a living room where the drapes were drawn, even at mid-day, according to Jim's father's recollections, whenever he called on his fiancée.

Recent studies suggest that almost 50 per cent of people diagnosed with bipolar disorder have issues with alcohol abuse and close to 60 per cent are addicted to illicit drugs. I have always been thankful that Jim never experimented with cocaine and other, more dangerous choices. Even so, Jim was always at risk of another relapse. At the time, I didn't understand the degree that alcohol could interfere with the efficacy of Jim's medication even when he was cautioned by his psychiatrist to drink sparingly. Perhaps the connection between his alcohol intake and his confrontational mood should have been more obvious to me. Admittedly, I wasn't helping matters much, already anxious, whenever Jim opened the second bottle of wine when we had guests for dinner, and he was the only one still drinking. Sometimes, I tried to keep up with him, so he would drink less. A sorry tale, to be sure, with both of us drinking more than we should.

I needed to set some ground rules. I was tired of being humiliated in front of others. I was tired of being anxious about the effects of excessive alcohol intake with his meds. I began to dread going to functions with an open bar. Although Jim denied that alcohol was a problem, I suggested that we ask his physician, Dr. David White whether he would conduct joint therapy sessions with us. Jim was resistant at first, but finally agreed that we should be setting some guidelines. It was a small step, but it paid off in the long run. If only Jim was as agreeable when it came to discussions about managing money.

On a Friday evening in September 2001, Jim's father came over for dinner at my request, to discuss some pressing financial matters. After a rather brief and very heated exchange on all sides, Jim accused us of ganging up on him. Instead of expressing regret for mishandling his financial affairs, Jim became very threatening, hurling a glass of wine at his father and throwing his dinner plate on the floor. Then he put his hands together in a religious pose, as if to absolve himself of any crime. We had experienced his volatile mood swings with religious connotations before, so his angry outburst frightened both of us. Although Jim may not have been experiencing full-blown mania, we felt that he still needed urgent care. Surprisingly enough, Jim agreed to be taken to the hospital for an evaluation, convinced that there was no need for us to be concerned about his unruly behaviour. As suspected, Jim was wrong.

After a lengthy intake process, Jim was admitted to the acute care ward of the Centre for Addiction and Mental Health late that night as an involuntary patient. Jim was angry, blaming me again for having him locked up against his will. Jim was also perturbed that he wouldn't be able to get in touch with the patient advocate until Monday to request a review of his status. He threatened to call the bank, and request to have his disability cheques deposited into his personal account, so I would no longer have access to his funds to pay the rent and other household bills. By now, my own anxiety level was sky high.

It was almost midnight, when I walked into our empty apartment and collapsed on the bed. Jim's recent actions created an even greater uncertainty in our relationship. And yet, I was unwilling to punish my husband for deeds when there was plenty of blame to spread around. I had to accept the reality that, somehow, I had failed him. As he and his brother put it so plainly, I should have known better and at the very least, taken some steps to stop Jim in his tracks.

If only that was possible.

While Jim was hospitalized, I spent the next few days going through Jim's drawers trying to find a paper trail of recent expenses to determine why Jim was in financial difficulty again. But there were no monthly statements, and no receipts, except for a P.O. Box at our local post office. In his Day-Timer, I found airline tickets for New York to celebrate our 28th wedding anniversary in December, as well as $100 tickets to see the hot new musical, *The Producers*. Hotel reservations had been booked at $700 a night, as well as a dinner at the price gouging new restaurant, Alain Ducasse at the Essex House. Like so many other travel arrangements, everything had been set in motion months ago. I made it clear to Jim when I visited him, that we were not going anywhere.

I contemplated, again, asking his psychiatrist to have Jim declared "financially incompetent" while he was still in the hospital, and then, filing for a continuance with the Office of the Public Guardian and Trustees, when he was discharged. But the onerous procedure was fraught with legal complications if Jim decided to contest it.

All the same, I was determined to impose some control over Jim's finances although it had always been a futile undertaking in the past. However, when I threatened to leave him, Jim reluctantly agreed to sign a document I had drawn up, witnessed by members of the medical staff, granting me continuing power of attorney in all financial and property-related decisions on his behalf.

In a letter written to his parents, Jim was remorseful:

You expect that your children will grow up, somewhat normally and become less of a burden and cause less stress as time goes by... I humbly apologize for my behaviour. I really don't think that anybody is going to come up with good reason for some of my actions...

Obviously, I am more than thankful to the support that I have received from Lembi – more than beyond the call of duty. I doubt very much if anyone could take the stress. Other issues like lies and breach of trust are very difficult to define and grasp.

Danielle Steel shared her own struggles with the disease in her heartfelt and courageous memoir *His Bright Light*, written about her son, Nick Traina, who died by suicide at the age of nineteen. She wrote about how hard it is to love someone with bipolar disorder and yet there is no choice but to stand by and provide the support they need.

In an email to my sisters, I expressed my own frustrations with a free-spending husband, writing: "I am only 55 years old and still in good health. Am I going to let Jim sabotage the rest of my life?" And yet, there was never any real threat that I might leave Jim, whether or not he kept his promises. How could I even think about walking out on him? His parents had never abandoned their son despite some very distressing times over the years. Besides, I was still in love with him. Even on the darkest days, the hope that there would be better days ahead was enough to keep the flames that first ignited our relationship from being extinguished.

Part IV

Fighting for Fairness Campaign
2000 - 2005

Chapter Eight – A Formidable Foe

Misbehaving badly

In all likelihood, there are no villains, only victims in this saga of mismanagement, intimidation, deception, corruption and fraud.

While I never had any intention of becoming "an accidental advocate," I couldn't let Jim down when he appealed his case to the tax court. He was counting on me, and there were others as well. I suspected there were hundreds, if not thousands of individuals, like Jim, unjustly denied the DTC.

I called my member of parliament (MP), Dr. Carolyn Bennett, a Liberal back-bencher representing St. Paul's, Toronto since 1997, and asked for her support. After successfully opposing a merger that saved Women's College Hospital in Toronto, the feisty family physician entered politics and quickly became an important voice for the disabled community. As a medical doctor, she also understood the incapacitating effects of a chronic, relapsing and remitting mood disorder. Dr. Bennett was certainly familiar with the difficulties that people impaired in their mental functions had accessing the DTC. As Chair of the Sub-Committee on the Status of Persons with Disabilities, she also had a responsibility to investigate discriminatory practices of the federal government's income support programs.

On March 23, 2001, I dropped off copies of my report for her committee members. The title was nothing to brag about though it described the contents well enough: *The Current Disability Tax Credit Certificate, Form T2201, its Impact on Individuals with Disabilities and Case Law*. I had done my homework and had every expectation that my submission would provide the compelling medical and legal evidence committee members needed to take necessary steps to protect the rights of all Canadians with disabilities. I also provided an extensive appendix pertaining to the challenges faced by Jim when trying to access the DTC.

In the meantime, I capitalized on the interest demonstrated in my husband's big win in court in June. I contacted major national health charities and together, we established the Coalition for Disability Tax Credit Reform.

At our first meeting in September, I assured the members of our fledgling organization that, "We will be successful because we share a commitment to do what is right... and there are too many people counting on us." I also noted that we were not going to allow ourselves "to get beaten down by the system." As it turned out, we would get beaten back more often than I care to remember, but never beaten down.

We began a letter writing campaign in earnest, urging Dr. Bennett and her committee to focus on the problems people were experiencing when trying to access the DTC. I was also contributing articles for newsletters, accepting speaking engagements, and urging everyone to write to their MPs, asking for their support.

With the assistance of Robert Currer, a close friend and a web master with extraordinary skills, I developed an Internet presence with www.disabilitytaxcredit.com. These were the early days of using social media as an advocacy tool. With Google already up and running, it was easy for others to find my website, most notably, civil servants who became my most frequent visitors.

When I met again with Dr. Bennett on October 11, she wasn't very optimistic as far as getting my submission onto the Sub-Committee's Fall agenda. At the time, concerns regarding the disability benefit provided by the Canada Pension Plan were an important priority. I was discouraged when my report ended up on the back burner.

Then, we got lucky. We got help from the enemy.

The timing could not have been better.

On October 19, the CCRA sent a form letter to 106,000 Canadians with disabilities raising questions about their entitlement to the DTC, and cutting them out of the program altogether:

After reviewing your file, we have determined that we do not have enough information to continue to allow your claim for the 2001 and future tax years... In order for us to re-evaluate your eligibility for the DTC, you need to send us a new Form T2201, Disability Tax Credit Certificate.... We appreciate your co-operation and understanding in this matter. We regret any inconvenience this review may have caused.

The unwarranted assault by the government on some of its most disadvantaged citizens was unprecedented. In order to continue to benefit from the modest tax measure designed to assist with some of their expenses, they were required to reapply for the DTC with a new, more restrictive application form. Adding insult to injury, they were expected to cover the medical practitioners' cost to complete the form, reported to be as much as $150 if additional information was required.

My friend Wilf, who had been given a lifetime exemption, was also targeted. A retired civil servant, he relied on a wheelchair because his body was horribly twisted out of shape by dystonia, a rare movement disorder. Wilf was on his way to Puerto Rico for the winter when the letter arrived at his doorstep.

I discovered soon enough, in a mysterious email from a government official who wished to remain anonymous, that the audit of the DTC program was inevitable. He claimed that there was a "cover-up of significant fraud and mismanagement" of the DTC program by senior staff at the CCRA. He also suggested that members of the medical profession were an accessory in the massive deception with "300,000 currently fraudulent claims."

We met a few weeks later in a darkened corner of the restaurant at the Sheraton Hotel in downtown Toronto. My contact shared a copy of his letter, dated July 5, 1999, to the former Minister of National Revenue, the Honourable Herb Dhaliwal. The lengthy letter provided the details of a massive fraud of more than $2 billion over ten years, that was "a huge embarrassment, largely of the Department's own making:"

It has already been proven, that only 20% of new claims actually meet the legislative intent... and 80% of new claims will continue to be endorsed by physicians who knowingly aid and abet the unentitled claimants... because there is no objective evidence requirements.

As your department had two years ago quietly absolved physician culpability by transferring all responsibility and (presumably) culpability, to the claimants themselves, physician endorsement has less legitimacy than before, i.e. no legitimacy... Physicians are hamstrung by their relationship with the patient, and few are prepared to risk the loss of business by refusing endorsement...

The result is, that fraud continues to go undetected and unchallenged because your officials... did not and do not wish to expose it, and themselves... Meanwhile 80% of those who benefit, have no right to it, either in the letter or the spirit of the law.

Minister Dhaliwal was replaced by the Honourable Martin Cauchon the following month in a cabinet shuffle. It took another two years for the government to act upon the complaint and send out letters to everyone under 65 who was receiving the DTC. There was no apology beyond a vague "regret" and certainly no admission of "its central role in this sorry state of affairs."

The uproar within the disability community was immediate. MPs across the country were besieged by their constituents. The Sub-Committee shifted its priorities, announcing that public hearings would be held with stakeholders to investigate a government determined to reduce its fiscal costs by targeting the disabled.

"Surely it is a response of a system that has gone a little mad," professed MP Wendy Lill, during the debate in the House of Commons on November 19, 2002:

When it comes to providing a relatively modest amount of additional financial support to a group of citizens who are by definition among the lowest incomes and most vulnerable in society... we tie ourselves into knots.

MP Lill, along with Dr. Bennett, championed the unprecedented unanimous vote, 243 to 0, the following day. I was literally sitting on the edge of the couch watching the vote on television. I was very pleased to see everyone on the front bench of the Liberal Party, including the Honourable Elinor Caplan, the Minister of National Revenue, also get up, one by one, for the "Yea" vote. Parliamentarians representing all political parties censured the CCRA and prevented the adoption of the restrictive eligibility criteria introduced a few months earlier by the Liberal government's Minister of Finance, the Honourable John Manley. The motion called on the government to overhaul the program and deal humanely with Canadians with disabilities. "The synergy of the disability community and our all-party committee has been a tribute to democracy…" Dr. Bennett had written in a letter to the editor of *The Toronto Star*. "We are now waiting for the government to act responsibly and compassionately."

Now, there was a challenge.

The CCRA was denying legitimate claims without a valid reason. Just as shameful was the blatant disregard for its own policies and procedures put into place to protect the interests of the taxpayer. Rejected applicants were not advised of their right to appeal an unjust decision. Nor were they advised of their right to documents filed by their doctors with the CCRA to assist with their appeal.

How was this possible?

The tax credit was originally designed to recognize undocumented, non-discretionary costs for people who were blind or confined to a bed or a wheelchair for a substantial part of the day. In 1986, it was expanded to include all Canadians with severe and prolonged mental or physical impairments. Previous guidelines for doctors, published in 1988, recognized people diagnosed with "schizophrenia, paranoid and other psychotic disorders" as qualifying for the DTC, noting that medically documented persistent symptoms can be "either continuous or intermittent." In 2000, the category of life-sustaining therapy was added.

DTC-related problems were identified as early as 1991 in a review by the Department of Finance when decisions about eligibility were made by medical advisors associated with the Department of Health and Welfare. In 1996, the Department of National Revenue assumed responsibility of the program. Instead of relying on doctor's descriptions of the disabling effects of the impairment, a revised application form, with check boxes, required a simple "yes" or "no" answer to a series of questions.

Unlike earlier efforts that recognized the unique burdens of those living with a serious mental illness, the determination of eligibility was now based on criteria that had no practical application in medicine. People living with a psychiatric diagnosis were automatically denied the DTC, if a doctor acknowledged that the "patient was able to think, perceive and remember" by checking the "yes" box. If the doctor checked the "no" box, the CCRA would follow-up with a so-called "clarification letter" which contained questions that defied common sense, including: "What percentage of the time during the day was your patient unable to think, perceive and remember?" Anything less than 90 per cent was reason enough to deny the DTC. Such an illogical assessment tool should never have been adopted in the first place. And yet, it remains in place to this day, discriminating against some of the most marginalized and oppressed citizens in our society.

The disability community was outraged by the requirement to re-qualify for the DTC, including Audrey Cole, a passionate advocate with the Canadian Association for Community Living, whose son had been approved for the DTC in 1987:

Has my son's file been destroyed? What additional information can we possibly supply? Nothing has changed... Our son hasn't suddenly learned to speak or to take care of his personal needs for toileting or nutrition, nor has he overcome the need for attendance by other people for every facet of his life. To suddenly imply that he's not supplied the authorities with sufficient information to remain eligible is arbitrary, insensitive, and totally rude.

Bill Casey, a Conservative MP representing Cumberland-Colchester in Nova Scotia, shared his concerns in the House of Commons about a constituent who had also lost the DTC. And then, he lost his life.

I was concerned that he was threatening suicide because of the frustration with the disability tax credit system... I talked to my staff about how often we hear this. They mentioned a person they knew who had committed suicide because of his frustration in not being approved for the disability tax credit because the government did not believe his doctors.

This man, Ralph MacEwan, suffered from chronic paranoid schizophrenia. The doctor said he was totally disabled. The reports were very clear, but the clerks at CCRA refused to accept the doctor's assessment and said Mr. MacEwan was not disabled and was completely able and okay. Out of frustration Ralph MacEwan took his own life.

A mother wrote a heart-felt letter to Minister Cauchon about her daughter:

Laurel Ann is mentally challenged due to a medical condition, hyperthyroidism. She is able to dress, feed and bathe herself. She is able to work part-time in a supported position in a Subway shop in Halifax. She cannot live alone, manage money, prepare meals, do laundry, shopping, pay her bills and all of the other things most of us take for granted.

Laurel Ann finds letters such as yours most upsetting, she is not able to understand what is being asked of her. Letters such as the one you sent on October 19th cause her a great deal of unnecessary stress.

Put yourself in her parents' place... can you imagine anyone saying their child is mentally handicapped or intellectually handicapped (it is no longer correct to call people retarded) if it were not true?

It is the most painful thing her father and I have had to deal with. People who work with the challenged adults of Canada may consider your letter a form of harassment.

Letters such as these urged MPs to take immediate action. And so, they did.

Dismay and dissatisfaction

On November 5, I received an anxious call from Bill Young, a research director with the Library of Parliament who was responsible for arranging committee hearings, recommending witnesses as well as providing members with briefing notes and drafting their reports. Mr. Young admitted that he could not remember, in 15 years, of an individual channelling a personal initiative into a parliamentary undertaking. He also explained that it was unprecedented for hearings to be organized in such an expeditious manner and so he needed assistance as far as compiling a contact list of witnesses. I was more than happy to comply with his request.

When I thanked Mr. Young in a follow-up email "for such good news" and the opportunity to participate in the planning process, he responded, telling me that, "It's always gratifying when things move forward (as opposed to sideways, or backwards)."

I had finally arrived at first base.

November 27 was a bitterly cold day as I walked from my hotel to the Parliament Buildings. The Canadian flag was flying high over the Peace Tower of the Centre Block, an invitation for all Canadians to take pride in their heritage. I still remember, so vividly, walking up the front steps and entering the main hall with its huge decorated Christmas tree. I felt very humble, nonetheless, empowered by the knowledge that an individual, an accidental advocate, could help set the wheels in motion to protect the disabled from government malfeasance. I had worked hard to get here and was suddenly overcome by the most wonderful feeling of belonging. As an immigrant whose parents escaped from the Russian advance into the Baltic countries during World War II, this was what democracy was all about. I was warmly welcomed by Mr. Young and others in a large committee room with several observers already seated in the chairs set aside for them. The television cameras were set up as the meeting was being recorded by CPAC. I was more than ready with my opening remarks:

Thank you, Dr. Bennett and members of the committee, for recognizing the urgency for a full review of the disability tax credit certificate that affects hundreds of individuals with mental illnesses who are being treated unjustly...

Mental illness is one of the least understood and least accepted of all illnesses. Individuals with mental illnesses remain among the most vulnerable members of our society. Unlike individuals with physical disabilities, they do not always have the intellectual capacity or the mental stamina to pursue their causes. For many, these illnesses are a source of shame and embarrassment. As a result, they are unwilling or unable to stand up for their rights when an injustice is done, and that's why I'm here today.

Len Wall, representing the Schizophrenia Society of Canada, also testified that the main problem facing government officials is the lack of understanding of the disabling effects of a serious mental illness: "From our experience, 100 per cent of new applications for this form from people with schizophrenia have been rejected." He was not alone.

Ed Pennington, CEO of the Canadian Mental Health Association wondered whether, "there has been a plot in the last few years to diminish the number of people who are eligible for the disability tax credit, and I don't know whether you have access to finding just where those missives came from and how they're implemented by clerks in the CCRA." He wanted to know, "how many millions of dollars could be saved on the backs of the disabled, just by virtually turning people down because of a phantom policy out there that's been imposed from on high."

Was it possible to accurately measure the crippling reality of living with a severe mental illness against the disabling effects of limited vision? Perhaps not. I did my best, trying to answer the question during my testimony the only way that made sense to me. I am legally blind in my right eye, so I understand the strict parameters to measure visual acuity for the determination of eligibility. And they are not nearly as stringent as the arbitrary threshold for mental impairments as I explained when I covered up my left eye:

If I lost the vision in my left eye, I would qualify for the disability tax credit. I can count all the people around the table. I can't make out the faces well enough to know exactly who they are, but I can distinguish between a man and a woman. I would have some challenges playing the piano, which I like to do, but I would have no problem shopping, cooking, taking care of myself, housekeeping, and hopefully, still have a job. I want to ask all of you, if you had a choice, what would you choose, being legally blind, where you can still function, or losing your mind?

On December 11, Dr. Bennett met with government officials for the first time. Apparently, she had stayed up until 3:00 am watching the CPAC tape of our testimony so she was ready for their responses to our concerns. She was also blunt with her own opinion of the application process for the DTC, telling them that, as a family physician, "This wasn't my favourite form to fill out before I got this new job."

As expected, the CCRA pushed back.

David W. Miller, Assistant Commissioner of its Assessment and Collections Branch, was quick to point out that he was unaware of any protests related to the dramatic policy changes that denied the DTC to previously eligible Canadians: "We have been using the form for five years, and we get 170,000 new applicants each year... and we've not had a single complaint or comment in that process." He didn't bother to share the shocking statistics that the vast majority of objections received by its Appeals Division since 1996, indicated a failure rate of 94 per cent of the original assessments denying the DTC, according to an Access to Information and Privacy (ATIP) request filed by MP Casey.

In an urgent letter to Minister Cauchon, Dr. Bennett had expressed "dismay and dissatisfaction" regarding the need for thousands of individuals to re-qualify for the DTC and subsequently, unjustly denied the tax credit. She asked him to send a letter of apology to all those who received the letter and provide the assurance that they would still receive the DTC in the 2001 tax year. When the Sub-Committee reconvened almost two months later, on February 5, 2002, with top officials from the Department of Finance and the CCRA, none of them had received a copy of her letter to the Minister. The cynicism in her voice was evident when she said, "So obviously, you haven't acted on the letter."

Senior bureaucrats would learn soon enough that you don't mess with Dr. Bennett, thanks to an unexpected source. *The Globe and Mail* reported on January 28, 2002, how Dr. Bennett incurred the wrath of Prime Minister Jean Chrétien by criticizing the lack of women in his new Cabinet during a television interview:

In a heated exchange during a caucus meeting of Liberal MPs and Senators, Mr. Chrétien pounded on the table and attacked backbencher Carolyn Bennett, a medical doctor, for her criticisms. He charged that she was damaging his reputation as a politician who had advanced women's issues.

"He beat up on Carolyn Bennett," said the MP, who did not want to be named... "It was just 'boom.' He just exploded," said another MP, who also did not want to be named...

Dr. Bennett returned fire, saying that she had spoken out in her role as chairwoman of the Liberals' women's caucus, MPs said.

Reports of the stormy caucus meeting led to the kind of notoriety that money simply could not buy. Dr. Bennett was featured by cartoonist Patrick Corrigan in *The Toronto Star*, trying to break through the glass ceiling while the PM thumbed his nose at her. There were other cartoons as well and Dr. Bennett became a media darling for taking a stand when it mattered most.

Clearly, Dr. Bennett was not about to be bullied by anyone. Not when she had spent hours listening to heart-wrenching stories from dozens of stakeholders about the mean-spirited actions by government officials denying a modest tax credit, essential to offset some of their extraordinary expenses. Not when her "urgent" letter had been brushed aside.

So, it was hardly surprising when Dr. Bennett expressed a certain degree of skepticism when addressing the senior officials from Finance and the CCRA:

We are thrilled to have with us today the people with all the answers as to why we're here. We trust you've been following with interest the hearings to date and have all the perfect answers for us.

Alas, there were no perfect answers. Instead, many of the responses to questions from committee members were incomplete, inaccurate, or misleading.

Kathy Turner, Director General, Benefit Programs Directorate for CCRA testified that major consultations with stakeholders in 1996 involved more than 900 associations and the Canadian Medical Association (CMA). The numbers alone were truly astonishing and consequently suspect. Unfortunately, the Sub-Committee was not provided with any documentation supporting her claims. To make matters worse, CMA's President, Dr. Henry Haddad had already raised troubling questions about the integrity of the consulting process in a previous committee hearing when he testified on January 29 regarding the extent of its role during government consultations.

The impression the Sub-Committee may have, is that the CMA has been consulted extensively and on an ongoing basis. In fact, these meetings, although productive - and I stress the fact that these meetings have been productive - have only occurred on an ad hoc basis. At best, our working relationship could be described as hit and miss.

Even more egregious was the outright false declaration made by Robert Dubrule, Senior Tax Policy Officer with the CCRA. When responding to the most controversial aspect of the determination of eligibility, that is, an individual must be markedly restricted at least 90 per cent of the time in a basic activity of daily living, he testified that the tax court rulings in several cases supported the inflexible guideline: "Given the jurisprudence in all of those cases involving the *Income Tax Act,* 'all or substantially all' has been interpreted as meaning 90 per cent."

The facts tell a different story. There wasn't a single case supporting the big lie. In fact, there were several cases, including my husband's that refuted his claim.

The testimony that day reflected an overarching need by senior government officials to protect the public purse. "Already the disability tax credit expenditures are close to $500 million, or something like that," stated Serge Nadeau, Director of the Personal Income Tax Division of the Finance Department. The bottom line according to Mr. Nadeau was that the government could not afford to be generous. "There's a trade-off that must be made among the fiscal cost, the fairness, and also, how easily it can be administered... Ninety per cent or 'all or substantially all' is a very clear test."

The clarity of Mr. Nadeau's argument was no doubt lost on the members when Ms. Turner claimed that, "Being disabled and being eligible for the credit are not entirely the same thing." In other words, some disabilities are more deserving than others when it comes to financial assistance from our government.

In March 2002, the Sub-Committee issued a scathing 44-page report, *Getting it Right for Canadians: The Disability Tax Credit*, calling for immediate action from the government to overhaul the DTC program. So, I was grateful to learn that my efforts to make a difference still mattered when I received the following congratulatory note from Mr. Young:

I work with a great group of MPs... (w)hen we can pull something like this report together, it is very gratifying. Even more so, because it doesn't happen every time. Of course, you must know that you played a very important role in pushing the issue forward and I really feel that a lot of the credit for keeping the politicians on side belongs to you. In many ways, this study and report is an example of Parliament doing what it's supposed to do and doing it well.

There was every reason to celebrate and I brought a bottle of Champagne to our next Coalition meeting. After all, we had made considerable progress in our efforts to ensure fair tax treatment for all

Canadians with disabilities. At least, that's what I thought. Looking back now, I realize that we were just getting started. It didn't take long to discover that the wheels of government turn very slowly, if at all. It could become very unnerving if the wheels started to move in reverse. And that's exactly what happened.

Back to square one

Incredible as it may seem, the government turned a blind eye and a deaf ear to the pleadings of not only the disabled community but also a bipartisan parliamentary committee. And it was all about the money and how much the government was willing to spend. On August 30, instead of acting on the recommendations of the Sub-Committee's report, the Department of Finance proposed amendments to the *Income Tax Act* to further tighten the eligibility criteria.

The CCRA had drafted a new application form that would make it more problematic to access the DTC for thousands of people who previously qualified, "if the effects of the impairment are episodic or intermittent." The cautionary statement on the cover page of the form was a blatant abuse of bureaucratic license discriminating against people living not only with mental illnesses, but also epilepsy and multiple sclerosis. The CCRA was essentially demonstrating its contempt for the Federal Court of Appeal's decision in my husband's case, *Attorney General v. James W. Buchanan 2002*, by refusing to accept the precedent setting legal opinion based on irrefutable medical evidence and the law.

Adding insult to injury, the government was planning to amend the legislation to prevent people requiring a gluten-free diet from qualifying for the tax credit. The problem was the unintended consequences of another recent unanimous decision by the Federal Court of Appeal in *Canada v. Ray H. Hamilton 2002*, allowing the DTC for a diabetic taxpayer who suffered from celiac disease. The digestive and autoimmune disorder required Mr. Hamilton to spend

188

"an inordinate amount of time identifying, finding and shopping for or otherwise procuring food" that he could safely eat. The problem facing the government was the additional financial burden to the DTC program if the flood gates, so to speak, were opened for everyone diagnosed with celiac disease. The only resolution was to close the loophole.

Dr. Bennett was furious. The rug had been pulled from under her by her own party elite. "I am extraordinarily disappointed by the Department of Finance," she said. "Everything that we have done to move this process forward in a democratic way has been undone."

It seems that our money was needed elsewhere.

While members of our Coalition were sending out hundreds of emails to elected representatives to stop all efforts to further restrict access to a modest tax credit for the disabled, federal finance officials were plotting and planning to ease the tax burdens of the rich and famous.

"Tax hit may be eased for Chagnons" was the headline of a report in *The Globe and Mail* dated September 23, 2002. A proposed amendment to the legislation would reduce André Chagnon's capital-gains tax by a whopping $180-million in the sale of his Vidéotron shares to Quebecor Inc.

The shameful irony was not lost on MP Casey who noted that the requirement to reapply for the tax credit was, "just another distasteful aspect of the government's ability to take this benefit away from the people that need it most. If those 58,000 Canadians all lose their benefits, the government will save up to $55 million - about the same as the price tag of one Challenger executive jet."

Once more, our collective persistence paid off.

MP Alexa McDonough, leader of the New Democratic Party (NDP) representing Halifax, called upon the government "to develop a comprehensive program to level the playing field for Canadians with disabilities, by acting on the unanimous recommendations of the committee's report to incorporate in a more humane and compassionate manner the real-life circumstances of persons with disabilities, and withdraw the proposed changes to the Disability Tax Credit, released on August 30, 2002." The subject matter was serious enough to set aside an entire day for debate in the House of Commons prior to voting on MP McDonough's motion on November 20, 2002.

Jim and I were in Ottawa that week, attending the Canadian Mental Health Association's annual conference. On the day of the debate, we sat in the gallery listening to elected representatives from across the country share their concerns. There were plenty of angry voices in the hallowed chambers of our democracy.

Dennis Mills, MP for Toronto-Danforth, described the "screw-up in revenue and finance" to disenfranchise thousands of Canadians with disabilities as "one of the most despicable things I have ever experienced in my 20 years on Parliament Hill."

Larry Spencer, MP for Regina-Lumsden-Lake Centre in Saskatchewan, reminded everyone that the request for fair treatment of all persons with disabilities was fiscally reasonable: "We are not talking about a real huge dollar hit on the federal budget. It is peanuts to the government and to the country... To slap these people in the face by not allowing them these kinds of benefits shows a callous and uncaring group of people who worry more about money than people."

Loyola Hearn, MP for St. John's West, was almost at a loss for words: "It is extremely hard to believe that we would try to take back from deserving people a minuscule amount that is so helpful to them but so little in relation to a budget, especially a budget that is administered by a department that brags about having an almost $40 billion surplus. It is unbelievable... With the little break that they get we are trying to withdraw it. It is terrible that the government would even think about such a thing."

MP Lill spoke on behalf of the members of the Sub-Committee: "We were all, bar none, stunned by the deep and calamitous response from all we heard from and we were ashamed... All of this is supposedly being done in the so-called public interest."

The unanimous bipartisan vote in the House of Commons the following day demonstrated that Canadians with disabilities deserved both the respect and support of elected representatives who were determined to protect their rights. But we were far from being home free. The next battle had just begun and threatened to sabotage any likelihood of achieving the objectives of fairness laid out in the Sub-Committee's report.

Who could have anticipated a vindictive enemy leading the charge against some of the most vulnerable members of our society?

In a nasty turn of events, the Department of Finance threatened the disability community with the loss of benefits. The backgrounder attached to its news release issued on November 29, referencing the Hamilton decision, stated the following:

In March 2002, the Federal Court of Appeal rendered a decision that would expand the eligibility for the DTC far beyond this policy intent... Such an expansion of eligibility would result in fewer resources being available to individuals with a severe and prolonged mental or physical impairment.

It was quite astounding, really, that a ruling in a taxpayer's favour could cause such alarm. Even more concerning was the ominous possibility that it would undermine the entire disability program in the country. If someone wins, why does someone else have to lose? Instead of looking for creative ways to incorporate the Hamilton ruling, the senior bureaucrats were prepared to deny the DTC to those already receiving it.

The NDP was not wasting any time and delivered 1500 letters to Prime Minister Chrétien, asking the Liberal government to abandon its proposed punitive amendments to the legislation. In its news release, MP Lill provided the following explanation for "Putting the Prime Minister on Notice":

191

These letters are a reinforcement to the unanimous vote in the House. Canadians are watching and will make sure that the Liberal government doesn't get away with simply waiting for an opportunity to sneak the changes through the back door.

This was not the first time that the government was faced with a significant increase of new DTC claimants. When the Cystic Fibrosis Foundation successfully lobbied the government, the *Income Tax Act* was amended in 2000 to include life-sustaining therapies.

The Hamilton case was different. The numbers were much bigger and, so it seemed, more ominous to the bean counters in Ottawa. The backlash from all sides led to consultations across the country with health charities. I was invited to the Toronto session held at the Royal York Hotel on December 13, where I put forward a proposal to limit the financial burden associated with the Hamilton case.

During a discussion following the meeting, Serge Nadeau, who had testified at the Sub-Committee hearings, was honest about his lack of enthusiasm for my recommendation since it relied too heavily on the integrity of the taxpayer to keep proper records. Nonetheless, he seemed to be impressed with my efforts and admitted that I wasn't anything like he expected. I didn't dare ask for an explanation when Serge added that I had a very high profile in Ottawa, which I interpreted as a back-handed compliment, if there ever was one. So, I was surprised when Serge asked if he could call me to discuss various issues related to the DTC.

My first impression of Serge was that he didn't dress like a government employee. He was a walking advertisement for a men's fashion magazine and I wondered if he was a regular customer of Harry Rosen at the Rideau Centre. Nor did Serge act like a self-serving distant bureaucrat, who might be more concerned with procedure or policy than with the people he served.

Serge and I were unlikely allies who became friends. Although we were worlds apart on some of our views, there was a mutual respect for each other's opinions. We spoke frequently over the phone discussing the Hamilton case and other concerns. I requested a copy of the trial transcript hoping to find an acceptable solution to break the impasse. I also suggested the need for a comprehensive review of DTC program, with all the major players at the table.

Stormy seas

Early in the new year, I was more than pleased to learn that Serge had followed up with my suggestion and set the wheels in motion to create such a committee. Although he wasn't in a position to divulge the details, Serge hinted that I would be delighted with the news in the upcoming Budget Speech in the House of Commons. I was flattered to receive a personal invitation from the Honourable John Manley, Minister of Finance (and Deputy Prime Minister) to attend the "tabling of the federal budget" and "reception to follow" on February 18, 2003. I couldn't help smiling at the notation of the "Cash bar" on the bottom right-hand corner of the invitation. Such restraint!

As much as I wanted to go to Ottawa, Jim and I would be back in California for our annual pilgrimage to Carmel for another Masters of Food & Wine event. Jim had been feeling pretty low all winter and I was hoping that an escape to a warmer locale would help alleviate his depressed mood. Of course, all the travel arrangements had already been made, much of it paid for, so there was no point backing out.

Serge had also expressed regret that I would miss such a momentous event, especially when Minister Manley wanted to meet me. Serge followed up later, providing details of the new Technical Advisory Committee on Tax Measures for Persons with Disabilities (TAC). A generous budget was already allocated for TAC, including $25 million for starters and $80 million annually to broaden the eligibility criteria for persons with disabilities. It was far more than I could have ever hoped for. When I was appointed to the new committee, Serge called again, to congratulate me: "Really, really happy that you accepted." In a follow-up email, he noted that the Minister's office was also delighted.

In retrospect, perhaps neither Serge nor the Minister's office should have been pleased with the appointment. In the first of many emails to Serge throughout the course of the next two years, I shared my concerns about early discord within the ranks. My position was always very clear. The money on the table was to improve access to the DTC, period. Instead, a few members were already sailing our ship into stormy seas as I was bracing myself for a very rocky voyage.

Dear Serge:

Some of the lines were drawn in the sand even before lunch on the first day... and the mandate of the committee has quickly moved from the relative safety of a protected harbour right out to sea... I hope we don't flounder out there too long, trying to take care of all issues related to disability and poverty...

I am also pleased to have the resources of Finance and the CCRA at the table. Nevertheless, I am concerned that the CCRA is already digging in its heels as well as being very defensive... they have never acknowledged that we have serious problems with the administration of the DTC.

At our next round of meetings, we were still spending an inordinate amount of time discussing broader disability and poverty issues. I was a relative newcomer to the cause, while others had been fighting for a better deal for the disabled for years, if not decades. Many were seasoned veterans of government consultations, revisiting old grievances. I was not only outnumbered but also, most certainly, outranked.

The membership of TAC was made up of professionals and leaders in their field, four lawyers, four executives of non-profits dealing with social policy issues, a child psychiatrist, a psychologist, a tax policy/economic consultant and me. I was not about to be intimidated by anyone, and redoubled my efforts reminding everyone that we had a clear mandate: "to make recommendations that would help the federal government improve the fairness of the treatment of persons with disabilities under the income tax system, taking into account, available fiscal resources."

Still, I had every reason to be worried that the allocated funds would end up elsewhere. I noted in my journal that Laurie Beachell, National Coordinator for the Council of Canadians with Disabilities had his own agenda, saying, "This is an advocacy initiative gone all wrong... and here we are discussing tax measures for persons with disabilities when so many are living in poverty."

I countered with, "This is an advocacy issue that has been hugely successful... we lobbied hard and the government listened to us." I stressed the urgency of our task, that our MPs were expecting us to fix the problems facing their constituents. I also mentioned that I was bringing boxing gloves to our next meeting.

Unlike others at the table, more often than not, I was spending seven days a week, forging ahead to help ensure a just result for people, like Jim, living with a severe mental illness. I noted my dilemma in a journal entry:

The DTC has become more and more of an obsession. I wake up several times at night and my thoughts are dominated by the DTC. So much to do. So many people to help. So many hurdles in the way.

When I got home from Ottawa, I bought a second-hand pair of bright red EVERLAST boxing gloves for $10. At our next meeting, my colleagues took notice when I reached into my sports bag for the gloves and put them on. There were no further disagreements. We quickly got down to the business we were asked to do.

Politics aside, there were still obstacles when trying to access information for various reports. Early on, I was put on notice for my efforts when my research revealed embarrassing details about the CCRA withholding information from disabled taxpayers about their appeal rights. I was also censured for contacting a senior government official without prior approval from the committee. In my defence, I claimed that following strict protocol guidelines was not working out for me. When asking for answers from our government representatives at the table, I had received erroneous information or questionable information or no information at all. If our committee was to fulfill its mandate, we could not allow the Department of Finance or the CCRA control our access to information.

I found myself apologizing to Sherri Torjman, Co-Chair of our committee for putting her in an awkward position of having to "rap my knuckles from time to time." And yet, I stood my ground, informing her in an email that I had "an obligation to thousands of Canadians with disabilities... to get as much done as I can... I am very conscious of the time... (and as a cancer patient), it's not a luxury that I can count on."

I also asked for an emergency meeting with Serge. We met for breakfast the following morning and I let him know, in no uncertain terms, that government officials were interfering (intentionally or not) with what I believed to be strictly committee business. I emphasized that our committee must remain independent in order to maintain its integrity. Otherwise, I was prepared to hand in my resignation. Serge followed up later in the day to assure me that I would have unfettered access to any information I needed for my reports.

Even so, Serge was not always on my side.

Liam's story

In another private meeting, I advised Serge that the parents of six-year-old Liam, living with type 1 diabetes (also known as juvenile diabetes), were unable to access the tax credit as well as the $1,600 Child Disability Benefit because they could not afford the $6,000 insulin pump. In one of the harshest, if not outright cruellest interpretations of the legislation, CCRA's policy statement was very specific as far as denying the DTC to children dependent on daily insulin injections:

In general, children with type 1 diabetes would qualify for the DTC under the life-sustaining therapy (LST) clause if (certain) criteria are met. Criteria: the child requires a continuous infusion of insulin via an insulin

196

pump AND this mode of insulin administration is a medical necessity (not a lifestyle choice). Individuals whose condition is controllable with daily injections of insulin do NOT generally qualify for the DTC, since the actual administration of the insulin injections would not require a total of 14 hours per week.

Liam lived in a remote fishing outpost on the west coast of Newfoundland. His father Roy was a welder and his mother Barb stayed home because of the intensive care required by her son. Liam was diagnosed with the more extreme "brittle" form of this disease, requiring his mother to check her son's blood sugar levels at least 8 to 12 times each day. In the middle of the night, while Liam was asleep, Barb would lance her son's little finger to draw enough blood for a reading in a glucometer. If necessary, without waking him up, she would feed him a Cheez Whiz sandwich, along with a juice box, to prevent a hypoglycemic episode during the night.

Barb couldn't understand why Liam had been denied the DTC for the 2002 tax year, considering she followed up with CCRA's request for additional medical reports. Unlike other children his age, her son was not able to feed himself without her supervision because of the complex system of carefully measuring blood sugar levels and counting carbohydrates to determine his daily food intake. Nor could she understand why she had to jump through so many hoops in the pursuit of justice, causing additional emotional stress on the family. When Liam was denied the DTC, she expressed her anger and frustration on her website, www.diabetesadvocacy.com.

I was livid! I screamed! I cried! I kicked the walls! What sort of idiots were making these decisions? Did they not read? Did they miss the part where Liam eats while he is asleep so that he doesn't die during the night of a hypoglycemic episode? What kind of medical expert could deny our claim?

Barb made a formal submission to our committee requesting fairness in the determination of eligibility for all children living with type 1 diabetes. While our committee supported her request, Serge was quick to express his concerns about the additional cost to the

197

program with approximately 20,000 children living with type 1 diabetes.

In the meantime, I reached out to Barb and assisted with her appeal to the Tax Court of Canada while she kept a progress report on her website, expressing her frustrations:

I still can't believe that I am having to fight in court to prove how much care and attention my child requires... As the date draws closer, my nerves begin to fray. I am still nervous about being in court but am incredibly confident in our case. I know we will win. It would take a lot to screw this up. The Gods are definitely on our side when it comes to type 1 diabetes and CCRA. We will win this fight--all of us!!

And so, we did.

After reviewing the evidence, the lawyer representing the Crown offered to settle the case out of court. It was a big win, but also bittersweet.

The amount under dispute was $7,000 for the 2000 to 2002 tax years, but Barb was denied the DTC for the two previous years, 2000 and 2001. In an extraordinarily parsimonious move, a senior official refused to deviate from standard operating procedure, advising Barb that, "The CCRA's policy... does not allow retroactive application of court decisions." She was also advised that Liam would have to start the process all over again and file a new application for 2003 since there was no requirement for the government to apply the court decision for future years, disregarding the fact that type 1 diabetes is a life-long, permanent condition.

From the outset, senior officials responsible for the public purse worried incessantly about the potential cost of each of our recommendations as we also reviewed policies supporting caregivers of persons with disabilities. At the same time, in an email, Serge noted that his colleagues were pleased with our efforts: "We feel that a lot of progress is being made on very difficult issues. Between you and me, we waited too long to set up this committee."

Our report, *Disability Tax Fairness,* issued in December 2004, led to major reforms of the *Income Tax Act* benefiting thousands of people previously unable to access the DTC. Major legislative changes also allowed for a better understanding of the difficulties faced by people living with mental illness. Just as important were the provisions allowing all children living with type 1 diabetes to access the DTC.

My $10 investment for the boxing gloves paid off handsomely, translating into millions of dollars more for people with disabilities. The Budget, tabled on February 23, 2005, by the Minister of Finance, the Honourable Ralph Goodale, was a huge personal victory. It had been just four years since my first meeting with Dr. Bennett in her office. Many of the 25 recommendations from our committee were adopted, either completely, or at least, to a significant degree. Taken together, tax relief for persons with disabilities and their caregivers had increased by $110 million for the 2005 - 2006 tax year.

While a member of TAC, I had recommended the creation of the Disability Advisory Committee (DAC) to act as a watchdog over the administration of the DTC. Quite honestly, I didn't trust the government to keep its commitments. I was pleased when the Minister of National Revenue, the Honourable John McCallum appointed me and other members of TAC to the new committee with its inaugural meeting on July 18, 2005. Unfortunately, our tenure was cut short soon after Stephen Harper and his Conservative party defeated the Liberals on January 23, 2006. Since then, many of the improvements have been all but lost. The new government was also very adept at subverting the parliamentary and legislative intent of the DTC by denying the tax credit to those who needed it the most.

The ultimate betrayal

My faith in government was shaken to the core by a breach of trust from an unsuspected source, a senior government official, whose actions essentially led to the defeat of the Liberal majority government.

In the Fall of 2005, after the close of the markets on November 23, Minister Goodale made a surprise announcement regarding tax matters related to dividends and income trusts. But there had already been heavy trading earlier that afternoon and share prices had risen sharply. When interviewed by CBC News, Minister Goodale denied that there had been any impropriety within his department. "We are always very careful and very discreet," he told reporters. "There was no leak."

On December 27, the RCMP announced that it was investigating the minister's office for engaging in insider trading. The United States Securities and Exchange Commission also announced that they would launch a probe. After an exhaustive 14-month investigation, my trusted confidant, Serge Nadeau, was charged with criminal breach of trust. The CTV News, in its online broadcast on February 16, 2007, provided the following stinging indictment:

It is alleged that he used confidential Government of Canada information for the purchase of securities which gave him a personal benefit, the Royal Canadian Mounted Police said in a statement. On November 23, 2005, the trading of income trusts and related stocks spiked hours before an anticipated announcement by then finance minister Ralph Goodale.

Minister Goodale was devastated to learn that one of his most senior financial advisors had violated a public trust, with the RCMP probe in the middle of the federal election campaign.

In an article published in *The Globe and Mail* on May 16, 2007, Minister Goodale admitted, "he was distressed that his reputation as an honest person of integrity and character was being questioned by others, noting 'this has been the single most painful period' in his political career. This is the first time I have regretted being involved in public life; it's just been sheer agony because the thing that matters most to me has been attacked."

Serge went on to teach economics at the University of Ottawa. He passed away on December 7, 2018 at the age of 62 from cancer. In his obituary posted online, his family remembers "his good nature and resilience, an easy laugh and a cheerful enthusiasm… and a sharp intellect. He loved friendly debating and the sharing of ideas."

I often relied on Serge for advice and support. I always trusted him to put the interests of our committee into perspective, to take into consideration how much a modest tax credit would mean to Canadians with disabilities in a country as wealthy as ours. And I was always prepared to listen as he weighed the pros and cons of our deliberations and how they would impact the bottom line of the public purse.

Despite Serge's missteps, his wife did not abandon him. Instead, the obituary notes that "Serge especially wants to thank Jocelyne for her patience and devotion. She was the love of his life."

I would also want to be remembered by Jim as being someone who always stood by him, perhaps not always patiently, but most importantly as, "the love of his life." There were, however, plenty of times when I was unsure whether our marriage was worth salvaging.

Part V

Handle With Care

Chapter Ten: A Precarious Balance

The seductive power of music to soothe the soul

My advocacy work was a distraction from the challenges on the home front, as Jim's mental health continued to be a concern. As a member of the Technical Advisory Committee (TAC), my travel allowance covered the cost of renting a car and driving to Ottawa, so Jim could join me. I was reluctant to leave him home alone when he was severely depressed. I dreaded the possibility that Jim might take his own life in a moment of desperation, when nothing mattered anymore.

We were in Carmel, California in February 2003, when I learned that Minister Manley's budget included an allocation of $25 million to create the committee that would be meeting in Ottawa on a regular basis for the next two years as well as additional funds to improve access to the DTC. As it was, I couldn't wait to get back home.

Although I had hoped that the trip would improve Jim's mood, his inability to shake off the doldrums only created greater anxiety about every aspect of the day. At breakfast in the morning, his hands were shaking so badly that he could barely hold his cup of coffee, and at dinner in the evening, he was drinking more than he should. I could hardly blame him, self-medicating with alcohol at the end of each miserable day. Jim had also been prescribed Seroquel (quetiapine), an anti-psychotic with sedative properties to help him sleep. Unfortunately, the initial dosage was too high since he was getting up in the middle of the night, and wandering around the room, in his sleep. I was terrified that he might leave our motel room in his boxer shorts so, I barricaded his side of the bed with our suitcases each night.

I was relieved when we finally boarded the plane and returned home. There was considerable self-pity in my last journal entry of our vacation, as I was tired of being just a caregiver, taking control of every aspect of our lives, even when my decisions exasperated Jim's already depressed mood. It would have been different if Jim appreciated my efforts, but he was irritable and downright snarky, when I had to remind him to take his meds. He just didn't seem to care anymore, not about himself, nor me. "Do I deserve more?" I asked myself. "Or will it be much the same, week after week and month after month?"

Once we were back home, Jim's doctor adjusted the dosage of Seroquel which greatly alleviated my own anxieties since our apartment had two balconies. If Jim opened the wrong door to leave the apartment for some unknown reason, the consequences could have been grave.

As in previous bouts of debilitating depression, recovery took time. And as his mood improved, Jim began to enjoy our trips to Ottawa. He was no longer afraid to leave the hotel on his own for fear of getting lost, and began going out for long walks during the day. He also discovered delightful restaurants in the ByWard Market and made all the dinner reservations. While sipping on a glass of wine, I would recall the day's discussions and Jim would provide valuable input. His support gave me the much-needed courage to stand my ground, whenever committee members would challenge my proposals. "After all," he asked, "is there anyone else in the room who knows more about the DTC than you?"

It has always been difficult to understand the dynamics of bipolar disorder, with its faulty network of neurotransmitters, and how it continued to dominate our lives, even when everything else seemed to fall within the bounds of accepted normal behaviour. And then, there would be the "ah ha" moment that would bring everything into perspective. Rather than shedding light onto the incomprehensible reality of Jim's penchant for surprises, it only deepened the mystery.

"I am going to be late," Jim muttered under his breath, while we were sitting at a traffic stop behind an endless stretch of cars for almost an hour.

It was mid-afternoon, the last day of September 2005, and we were more than half-way home to Toronto from Elliot Lake, after the annual dinner hosted by Rio Algom for its former employees and retirees.

"Late for what?" I asked.

"For an opera, the world premiere of *Doctor Atomic*."

The flagman had already warned us that the road work would take at least an hour, before traffic could resume. I advised Jim that we would be home in plenty of time for him to get changed into something more suitable for the opening night performance by the Canadian Opera Company.

"The opera," Jim explained, "is in San Francisco tomorrow night. I have a plane to catch."

While Jim was stable on his meds, there was still an undercurrent of manic manipulation going on, in secret, to attend the modern opera by contemporary American composer, John Adams. The production described the stress and anxiety leading up to the first-ever, test detonation of a nuclear weapon in Los Alamos, New Mexico.

I was trying my best to keep a tight lid on my own explosive emotions, when I demanded to know how long Jim planned to keep me in the dark. Besides, what would blowing up, then and there accomplish, considering Jim admitted that he hadn't thought about it? Now, as I try to recall the conversation, Jim conceded that he might have called me when he arrived in California, or perhaps not. After all, he only planned to be away for a few days.

Jim had executed every detail of his trip very carefully to keep costs to an absolute minimum, using loyalty points to cover travel costs and a hotel stay for one night. He was catching the red-eye to Vancouver and transferring to a flight for San Francisco. He certainly wasn't splurging on the price of the ticket either. By spending only $10 for the standing room area behind the orchestra seats on the main floor, Jim believed that he was demonstrating some restraint.

Who was he kidding?

That was when Jim was promoting his own dream of producing an opera, with a query letter to Peter Herrndorf, the President and CEO of the National Arts Centre in Ottawa. I should not have been surprised by Mr. Herrndorf's response:

Many thanks for taking the time to write and share your idea... You inquired about the feasibility of commissioning an opera, and suggested that the Halifax explosion of 1917 would make an excellent dramatic subject. I think it's a wonderful concept and I'd be delighted to pass it along to Richard Bradshaw (General Director of the Canadian Opera Company).

Nothing was more sacrosanct than Jim's love for opera. Back in November 2000, I didn't discover his plans for a five-day cultural tour to Washington D.C. until a few weeks prior to his departure. The trip had also been planned in secret long before the house of cards came tumbling down. I was reluctant to say anything because of the brief notation in my journal while he was away that, "Jim has been much kinder and more considerate in recent months." And sometimes, that's all that mattered.

We were the lucky ones. We followed the science, as imperfect as it was when we met in New York, 50 years ago. How sad and unfulfilled Jim's future would have been, if he had been left to rely on his own interpretation of mania, back in February 1973. What if he had refused medical treatment with heavy-duty psychotropic drugs that allowed him to reconnect with the real world?

Jim doubts very much that he would be alive today, if he had not been taken into police custody and hospitalized against his will. After all, whenever Jim was on top of the world, so to speak, he was not aware that he was ill. Would I be alive today, when Jim threatened my life, while believing that he was on a mission for God? Such musings are frightening, indeed. Yet, these are the same fears that so many families are facing, while struggling to find appropriate care and treatment for loved ones when we have a critical shortage of acute care psychiatric beds in our general hospitals.

In *An Unquiet Mind*, Dr. Kay Redfield Jamison speaks out against the use of the more popular diagnostic term bipolar I disorder, instead of the historic designation to define her own medical condition, since it "obscures and minimizes the illness it is supposed to represent." As a person and a patient, she finds that, "The description, 'manic-depressive,' on the other hand, seems to capture both the nature and seriousness of the disease I have, rather than attempting to paper over the reality of the condition."

In the early days, there were so many questions and very few, if any, answers. I discovered shortly after meeting Jim, that it was impossible to keep up with someone in a manic state. I had no idea that his incredible energy and relentless drive, as well as his unbridled enthusiasm and grandiose self-esteem, were symptomatic of a mental illness. He believed that we were destined for greatness, if we just followed our dreams. Why should I not have believed him? I didn't know any better. Regardless, what could I have done, if anything, to stop him, once he started to go off the rails?

Even now, the symptoms can be ever so subtle, or carefully controlled, especially if Jim seems so "normal" otherwise. That certainly was true with Jim, who could be lucid and rational, even logical, during a manic episode. When Jim was not "mad" enough to be committed, it did not necessarily mean that he was sane enough to lead a perfectly "normal" life. More often than not, I excused his indulgent behaviour, and indiscretions that lacked good judgment, as symptoms of the disease, a medical issue, not to be confused with a moral or character flaw.

I now realize that Jim's bipolar disorder, after the major setback in 1990, was never properly under control with medications, certainly not 100 per cent. But what did that mean? While Jim has always had a great deal of restraint in some areas, it has been less so in other instances. Sometimes, there was no rhyme or reason for his actions. Despite the advances in neuroscience, it is still impossible to unravel the DNA and RNA molecules and pick out the offending bits and pieces that affect his moods and determine his behaviour.

Although we have excellent medications to treat episodes of acute mania and severe depression that have provided some sense of normalcy in our lives, they haven't alleviated all of the symptoms. Certainly, there has been less drama in our lives than the earlier years. But, the challenges of dealing with the fallout of unpredictable mood swings has remained a constant throughout much of our marriage.

After Jim's hospitalization in 2001, with the addition of new meds, our lives settled down to some degree, but not entirely. Even when Jim's mental state appeared to be relatively stable, when he seemed so "normal" otherwise, how could I know whether he was plotting another getaway? Even when the signs and symptoms of mania, or the lesser destructive hypomanic behaviour, were obvious, there was nothing I could have done to stop him. Not when his plans were so carefully executed, in secret, leaving nothing to chance.

In October 2006, we decided to drive to New York City to attend Anthony Minghella's stunning production of *Madama Butterfly* that had received rave reviews. Jim had also suggested that we head north along the coast to Boston for a day or two before going home. That was fine with me. Boston was one of my favourite cities and I was more than agreeable to go along with his plans.

We had checked into our hotel and spent the rest of the afternoon walking around in downtown Boston when I suggested that we look for a restaurant for dinner.

"It better be fast," said Jim.

"Why is that?" I asked, checking my watch. It was just after 6:00 pm.

"Because I have tickets for the Barbra Streisand concert at 7:30 pm."

I stood there, I don't know for how long, looking at Jim, who was very pleased with himself, being able to surprise me with tickets to the sold-out concert. We managed to squeeze ourselves into a crowded pub for a quick bite and a glass of wine before heading over to the arena where Streisand would be appearing, as part of her first tour in more than a decade.

And there I was, one of the luckiest people in the world, along with thousands of concert goers willing to shell out hundreds of dollars for tickets. Of course, it goes without saying that we had excellent seats.

Streisand wowed the audience during the two-and-a-half-hour show, complete with a 58-piece orchestra, though she relied on a large teleprompter for the lyrics, in case she might forget a line or two. What struck me the most, was that she too, was getting older. Streisand at 64, her neck was sagging a bit, like mine, and she had the same age spots on her hands, easily seen on the large screens above us. And when her feet were sore, Streisand kicked off her shoes as she sang, "Don't rain on my parade."

There was no point chastising Jim for leaving me in the dark months ago when tickets for the concert went on sale. Not when he was marching to the beat of his own drum, and as usual, with me just tagging along.

One day, when I was home alone, the phone rang. The call was for Jim. I explained that he was not available but I would be happy to take a message. An exuberant travel agent explained that she was calling from the Playbill Travel Agency, and apologized about the changes in our flight to Tahiti the following month.

"Tahiti?" I asked in bewilderment.

There was a long pause. Nothing should have surprised me any more.

"Am I speaking with Jim's wife?" she asked cautiously.

"Yes," I responded quickly, not wanting to let on that I knew nothing about the trip. And so, I suggested that she send the details to Jim's email address and he would call her if there were any further questions.

I certainly had plenty of questions to ask Jim when he got home. I had no idea that Jim had booked a cruise that would take us to some of the most gorgeous islands on the planet in French Polynesia, including Bora Bora and Moorea.

Of course, Jim was annoyed that the cat was out of the bag. He had hoped to surprise me on Valentine's Day with the details. This was no ordinary sojourn at sea on *M/S Paul Gauguin*. The travel agency was presenting "Broadway on the High Seas," with many of its brightest stars performing each evening. For Jim, it was the ideal blending of a cruise in paradise with some of the biggest names in the business.

How could I be angry at him? Jim was not about to divulge the cost of the cruise but felt justified, when making the decision without consulting me. After all, his father, who had passed away the previous year, had left him a small inheritance. Why would I object if he was picking up the tab? Why indeed?

Music has always played an important role in Jim's life. When we met, Jim had already amassed a considerable record collection. His most notable recordings included dozens of complete opera scores, at least a hundred works of classical musicians, and many of the musicals staged on Broadway. There was also a respectable collection of jazz, folk music, and so much more.

I have often wondered if there is a specific link between music and the bipolar brain. Studies have shown that music improves overall brain function, by stimulating the release of dopamine, the feel-good neurotransmitter that contributes to pleasurable experiences. For Jim, it was never just about listening to a record or CD. There has always been an affinity to music that I had never seen before, as if the vocal or orchestral arrangements of a song, musical or most notably opera, transcended his very being and transported him into another realm altogether.

While I am deeply indebted to Jim for enriching my life, I have never shared his passion for Richard Wagner. Not that Jim didn't make the effort, with tickets to a performance of his favourite opera, *Parsifal*, while we were in Chicago to celebrate our 40th wedding anniversary.

Nor have I interfered with his support for opera companies on both sides of the border, except for cancelling charitable contributions on more than one occasion, but only when his impulsive manic expression of generosity exceeded his financial means. However, I was powerless to stop his purchases of records, videos and CDs, as much as I agonized over my inability to stem the flow of music bought online that has crossed our threshold.

Life became more complicated when Jim's plans to attend the week-long Bayreuth Festival in Germany coincided with another cancer diagnosis. Despite the ever-present health challenges facing both of us, we were survivors. That being said, I was not willing to put Jim's life on the line when I discovered a small lump in my breast while we were on vacation. Instead, I was willing to make some sacrifices of my own.

We were celebrating my 66th birthday at the end of May 2012, driving across the United States to the Outer Banks in North Carolina. Jim and I had fallen in love with the rugged beauty and the fragile landscape of the barrier islands when we visited previously in 1999. And so, we were looking forward to spending an idyllic week at a hotel set back in the dunes overlooking the Atlantic Ocean.

I woke up early the first morning for a walk along the desolate beach, hoping to find some unusual shells to take home to our grandchildren. While applying a generous amount of sunscreen over my chest area, I felt the small lump, the size of a pea, and just as firm to the touch. I kept rubbing my finger over it, as if I could make it disappear.

When I returned from the beach, Jim was still asleep, and I was not about to wake him up. Whatever my fears, I was not going to spoil our vacation by having him worry about a small mass that could very well turn out to be a benign cyst. So, I said nothing to Jim, not then, and not even when we got home. There was no point worrying him or anyone else for that matter, not until I had some results. As it turned out, the biopsy was positive and the date for surgery was set for the same day in early August that Jim was leaving for Germany.

I was caught in an impossible situation.

Jim had been on a ten-year wait list, just to purchase the tickets for the prestigious Bayreuth Festival in Wagner's home town. Every year, he had sent in his application for tickets, hoping that his order would be accepted. When he was finally advised that tickets were available, it was a matter of arranging air and rail travel, as well as hotel accommodations. If Jim had to cancel his trip, he would have to start the process all over again. So, I said nothing and had my cancer surgery rescheduled for a date when Jim would be back home.

No one, besides my doctor, was aware of the conundrum I was dealing with. I was afraid that the shock of another cancer diagnosis might trigger yet another acute manic episode in Jim. I could not let him leave the country under such circumstances. No point having both of us back in the hospital at the same time again. Besides, I was betting on the fact that delaying surgery for a few weeks was not a significant factor while weighing the odds on both sides. Of course, I didn't tell anyone else either, not my children, nor my parents, nor any of my friends. I was afraid that word might somehow leak back to Jim. I was not prepared to take the risk, since I was far more stressed out about Jim travelling alone in a foreign country, than my own predicament.

Fortunately, my hunch was right. The tumour was a common, infiltrating ductal carcinoma found early enough, with no spread of the dreaded disease to other tissues or lymph nodes. After four weeks of radiation treatment, I was home free. And Jim was well. Our love affair had sustained another crisis.

The timing couldn't be better for a new lease on life. More than ever before, I would need all of my strength and Jim's support, as the tide began to turn against the very people who had benefited from the early years of my efforts to improve their access to the DTC.

Part VI

Fighting for Fairness Campaign
2014 - 2023

Chapter Ten - Here We Go Again

Resurgence of discriminatory practices

Accessing the DTC should not be a crap shoot. And yet, with the government's over-zealous approach to cut costs, it would only get worse. In fact, we hadn't seen anything yet. As distressing as it was to see Canadians with disabilities denied the DTC on questionable grounds, no one was prepared for the unprecedented action by the CRA to thwart justice by closing the doors to professional and legal assistance to those who wished to dispute a decision rejecting their claim.

How did it ever come to this?

Like employees of heartless insurance companies following orders, civil servants, with no medical training, were sending form letters rejecting claims without providing a relevant explanation for their decisions. That's hardly surprising since there has always been a serious lack of literacy among assessors, as far as interpreting the information provided by doctors and other health practitioners completing the application forms and follow-up questionnaires. To make matters worse, the CRA staff had unfettered discretionary power to say "no" to thousands of legitimate claims regardless of the medical evidence. And why would they do that? Why indeed? And yet, the facts speak for themselves. It's no secret among tax lawyers that the CRA has always counted on a tax system too complicated or expensive for most people to appeal a bad decision.

It was even more egregious when the CRA denied the DTC to Barbara Cochrane when there was no reason to do so. Despite her disability, she found the courage to fight back, and her case underlines how difficult it has become for people living with a mental illness to access justice. Although Ms. Cochrane was eligible for the DTC in 2010, she was denied the tax credit in 2016 when asked to reapply even though the two claims were identical and completed by the same doctor. In *Cochrane v. The Queen 2017*, Judge Bruce Russell recognized that Ms. Cochrane met the legal test for "all or substantially all of the time" due to her severe depression and anxiety. He accepted her argument that, "copying of the earlier certificate was done by Dr. MacDonald in a quest for administrative expediency in view of unchanged circumstances." Judge Russell noted that there was no reason for the assessor to reject a claim that had been previously allowed.

Needless to say, there was more work to be done to level the playing field for people severely impaired in their mental functions.

An unexpected call from the Governor General's office on November 2, 2015 would draw me back into the battleground in a renewed fight for fairness. I was being awarded the relatively rare Meritorious Service Medal, created in 1991, to recognize individuals, "for exceptional deeds that bring honour to their country," noting that:

Lembi Buchanan played a crucial role in income tax reformation by creating the Fighting for Fairness campaign. Through her intense lobbying, the need to broaden the eligibility criteria for the Disability Tax Credit received national attention, and led to persons with mental and episodic disabilities benefitting from the federal tax credit.

Jim, Jonathan and Larissa were present at the awards ceremony held at the Chan Centre in Vancouver. My children never complained about the hours I spent assisting others. Their only reward was the applause when their mother was recognized for her efforts to make a difference in the lives of others. Jim also had new business cards printed for me with the letters MSM after my name.

Despite the recognition for my work, I can't say there was much enthusiasm left to pick up the boxing gloves against an old adversary that kept changing the rules, sometimes, from one year to the next. Did I have the stamina to start all over? I had to admit that I wasn't always very good at compartmentalizing my life or managing my priorities. All too often, I was worn out by the end of the day. Then, there were the sleepless nights when addressing the feelings of helplessness and hopelessness that so many faced. I simply couldn't understand how our government could be so crass, so cruel, to renege on its commitment for equitable treatment of all Canadians with disabilities. And so, it was my job, once again, to call up the troops.

The renewed fight for fairness would be as nasty as anything else I had previously experienced. This time the devious tactics to restrict access to the DTC were carefully crafted and widely enacted. The CRA not only broadened the target group, but also doubled down in a deliberate attempt to deceive our elected parliamentarians during Question Period in the House of Commons.

There was nothing new about government taking advantage of disabled Canadians when it was all about keeping a lid on rising costs. The CRA continued to find surreptitious means to deny the benefit to eligible individuals to limit the number of people accessing the DTC.

Why?

I have asked that question a hundred times, no, a thousand times. But it was always about the money, regardless of which party was in power. Besides, the stakes were much higher now. The DTC not only reduced the taxable income for individuals with disabilities, but it had also become the gateway to important federal income support programs including the Child Disability Benefit (worth up to $2,730 in 2016) and the Registered Disability Savings Plan (RDSP).

The Conservative government introduced the RDSP in 2008, a tax-sheltered savings plan to help provide future financial security for Canadians with disabilities. Eligible individuals could access up to $3,500 annually in matching government grants and a $1,000 bond. However, when these individuals were asked to reapply for the tax credit, and then rejected, they not only also lost the DTC, but also their RDSP. By 2018, the CRA had closed the accounts of 4,503 disabled individuals and recovered $26 million in contributions, as if their need for financial support, somehow, was never legitimate.

These individuals never abused the system. These individuals never broke the rules. Indeed, there was no rationale to penalize Canadians with disabilities, even those who were no longer deemed to be eligible for the DTC. Instead of benefitting from a gift that keeps on giving, these individuals were required to repay all government contributions allocated in the previous ten years.

The Department of Finance was on a mission to balance the budget. And this time, decisions at the highest levels of government would have devastating consequences for thousands of Canadians with disabilities for years to come.

Starting in 2012, senior CRA executives were asked to target $4 billion in permanent savings for the Agency. We don't know if they received performance bonuses for their efforts, but it became more difficult to access the DTC. The revised application form, with its inflexible 90 per cent guideline, was a major barrier for individuals living with medical conditions where a mathematical model was not a suitable measurement of disability.

"How can they do that?" demanded the late Honourable Donald G. H. Bowman, during a phone call on March 10, 2016. The former Chief Justice of the tax court had retired from the bench in 2008 after an exemplary career. However, he had remained active, addressing law students and dispensing judicial wisdom based on two principles that guided him throughout his career: ordinary fairness and common sense.

Peter Weissman and I reached out to Justice Bowman for a better understanding of the logistical hurdles that left so many people behind. A partner with Cadesky Tax in Toronto, Peter was the Co-Chair of the former Disability Advisory Committee (DAC) that was disbanded by the Conservative government on February 6, 2006. We shared concerns about CRA's glaring disregard not only of its own policies and procedures but also of numerous tax court rulings that provided guidance as far as interpreting the legislative intent of the *Income Tax Act*.

The CRA was also defying the 1998 Supreme Court of Canada's decision in *Rizzo & Rizzo Shoes Ltd.* The ruling noted that, "benefits-conferring legislation... ought to be interpreted in a broad and generous manner. Any doubt arising from difficulties of language should be resolved in favour of the claimant."

During our call, Justice Bowman was quick to criticize the senior staff at the CRA, calling them "an arrogant bunch" as if taxpayers are "crooks and cannot be trusted." He noted that the administration of our tax system was unfair, inefficient and not accountable to anyone, claiming that "the Department of National Revenue routinely ignores certificates by doctors that a patient has a severe and prolonged impairment." He also explained that, "Interpreting 'all or substantially all of the time' as being at least 90 per cent may be a convenient measure for the CRA but it simply doesn't apply in all circumstances. It is misleading. It is not a reasonable assessment. There is no logic to it."

The collective abuse of CRA's own mandate for fairness by senior officials was truly shocking, when its legislative branch had already acknowledged in a policy document that, "the words 'substantially all' cannot be rigidly interpreted as referring to a specific percentage in all cases." Without a doubt, there was a need to assist taxpayers to navigate the Byzantine application and appeal process where the odds were stacked against them.

The blame game

CRA's heavy-handed tactics spawned the growth of a profitable industry of DTC consultants, operating on a contingency fee basis. Their work is highly specialized, requiring detailed knowledge of the tax credit, as well as related policies, administrative procedures and court decisions. There has never been any doubt that they provide an indispensable service to Canadians with disabilities. Instead of billing their clients on an hourly basis, these companies charge a percentage of the refund of successful claims.

There is nothing mysterious about contingency fees. They are the mainstay of personal injury and wrongful death law suits, ensuring that individuals have access to justice without paying any legal fees until their claims are settled. Many of these claims are complicated to process and may take years to resolve. The same can be said for applications for the DTC that also drag on for months, and much longer, if a decision denying the tax credit is contested. Relying on DTC consultants willing to work on a contingency fee basis has been the best possible solution for those without the financial means to hire accountants and lawyers at hefty hourly rates.

Nobody denies that the industry got off to a rocky start. Dubious business practices and aggressive marketing tactics would dominate the conversation regarding the legitimacy of unlicensed tax consultants for years to come. As one would expect, the CRA followed up on early allegations of fraud and deceit that led to investigations of the principals of two businesses.

Akiva Medjuck, President of the National Benefit Authority (NBA) in Toronto was in trouble with the CRA right from the outset. He was familiar with the work with the Technical Advisory Committee that led to major reforms in 2005. One of the amendments to the *Income Tax Act* allowed retroactive claims going back for ten years, which could create substantial tax refunds for disabled individuals.

The math was obvious. Contingency fees ranging from 20 to 30 per cent would net the company $4,000 to $6,000 on a $20,000 refund to support its business model, which also included covering the administrative costs of the time spent on failed applications.

In a joint investigation in February 2011, *The Toronto Star/CBC* reported that NBA was paying Mr. Medjuck's brother-in-law, Dr. David Neger to complete application forms for clients who did not have a family physician. The recent graduate of the Sackler School of Medicine in Israel was not licensed to practice medicine in Canada, and the CRA subsequently demanded refunds from taxpayers if their claims were certified by Dr. Neger.

NBA cleaned up its act and carried on, launching an aggressive advertising campaign and becoming the country's largest DTC service provider. When speaking with CBC reporter Jennie Stiglic, Mr. Medjuck was unapologetic about the 30 per cent commission on successful claims: "If there wasn't a need for this service, then we wouldn't be talking right now. But obviously, there's a huge need."

The CRA also investigated J & J Canadian Grants Company in Winnipeg. According to the sworn information required to obtain a search warrant, three business partners, Jose Diogo, Jim Kussy and John Lopes, along with Dr. Clarita Vianzon, participated in a scheme to secure tax refunds based on "false or deceptive statements." The CRA alleged that the company's clients were routinely directed to Dr. Vianzon, who charged from $50 to $100 to complete their application forms. According to the search warrant, at least 262 were issued refunds, valued in total at $2.8 million. The applications for another 700 individuals were frozen. In April 2013, the four principals pleaded guilty to charges of fraud. Each was fined $89,000 and given conditional jail sentences, ranging from 6 to 18 months. The CRA took steps to recover the refunds received under this scheme, unless the company's clients were able prove their eligibility through an independent medical practitioner.

Although there were no further reports of illegal activities, the CRA never stepped up to the plate to assist individuals with the application process. Instead, the Agency maliciously branded legitimate businesses, the only resource for many people who had nowhere else to turn, as "promoters." Granted, there has never been a direct connection made with the unscrupulous male cartoon character depicted on CRA's website and DTC consultants providing services to disabled Canadians. But then again, the warning could not be more explicit, suggesting that these businesses may be involved with shady activities:

"Promoters" are individuals or corporations who promote or sell schemes that seek to break or bend the rules of the Canadian tax laws. These promoters deliberately make false statements to assist their clients in tax cheating, all the while obtaining a financial benefit.

Negative news reports of predatory practices by some companies, allegedly charging excessive contingency fees, just added more fuel to the fire. Concerns raised by elected representatives ultimately led to parliamentary hearings with Conservative MP Cheryl Gallant of Renfrew-Nipissing-Pembroke leading the charge. On November 5, 2012, she introduced her Private Members Bill C-462, the "Disability Tax Credit Promoters Restrictions Act" to restrict the fees charged by companies assisting disabled Canadians.

While the ostensible purpose of the legislation was to protect people from unethical business practices, there were no supporting documents that anyone had been swindled. Sure, there were a few media accounts about concerns related to excessive contingency fees, reportedly as high as 40 per cent, but no proof of wrongdoing. Also, no one disputed the overall success rate of accessing the DTC with the assistance of these service providers, which was significantly higher for people with complex medical conditions, than attempting to access the elusive tax credit on their own. Nor was there any doubt as far as allocating blame for the rapid growth of such a lucrative industry. It lay squarely on the CRA for failing to ensure fair treatment for all Canadians with disabilities.

Dr. Karen Cohen, CEO of the Canadian Psychological Association, was certainly aware of the problems facing people living with mental illness, who were denied the DTC. When appearing before the House of Commons Standing Committee on Finance on May 7, 2013, she stressed, "… it is important to address what might be the underlying cause driving the use of promoters. If it is indeed the lack of clarity for taxpayers and health practitioners, then the criterion certificates themselves should be revised to enhance the fairness of assessments."

Dr. Gail Beck, a child psychiatrist representing the Canadian Medical Association, also blamed the CRA: "Why do vulnerable people need to go to these promoters in the first place? We suggest the disability tax credit form be revised to be more informative and user-friendly for patients. Form T2201 should explain more clearly to patients the reason behind the tax credit and explicitly indicate that there is no need to use third-party companies to submit the claim to CRA."

No one was more familiar with the problems disabled Canadians faced when going head-to-head against the CRA than Akiva Medjuck since his company was processing hundreds of applications every week. He also testified before the finance committee, stating the obvious: "We all know taxation issues are by nature complicated. The DTC is no exception. Canadians with disabilities need to have someone in their corner with the expertise and resources necessary for representing their interests."

Paul, who suffered from numerous severe and chronic medical conditions, said it best in his email to me: "The evil government itself created the need for disability tax credit specialists." Paul had been eligible for the DTC since 2001 but when he was asked to reapply for the tax credit in 2015, the CRA pulled the plug on his benefits. Paul was distraught. There was a great deal at stake, not only the loss of the $1,500 annual tax credit but also $30,000 in government contributions to his RDSP. A lawyer had quoted a $60,000 fee to fight CRA on his behalf in tax court. Instead, Paul got in touch with Canada Consultants (pseudonym) and acknowledged that the $800 fee, 20 per cent of his refund, "was worth every penny."

By the time the Senate Standing Committee on National Finance held hearings on MP Gallant's Bill C-462 on April 1, 2014, the situation facing the disability community had become dire. In his attempt to cut spending and balance the books, Stephen Harper's Conservative government had dramatically reduced the size of federal public service in 2012, creating a backlog in disability claims across several agencies, including Veteran's Affairs Canada. In October 2013, the CRA closed its service counters at tax centres across the country.

There was nowhere else to go for assistance when the CRA was imposing stricter eligibility guidelines to access the DTC, except to companies willing to work with their clients on a contingency fee basis to achieve a just result.

While there was no evidence that taxpayers were being exploited by DTC consultants when assisting them with their applications and appeals, there was plenty of criticism of the practice within the disability community. In his weekly column on tax matters in the *Financial Post*, dated June 7, 2019, Jamie Golombek, reported MP Gallant's outrageous claim that applying for the DTC was a simple matter: "It only takes a few minutes and doesn't justify the thousands of dollars that promoters are scooping into their coffers." And yet, in a previous column, dated December 14, 2018, Mr. Golombek described how qualifying for the DTC was "an uphill battle for many."

Despite efforts to discredit and undermine an unregulated industry of DTC consultants, these companies continued to play a vital role ensuring access to the tax credit and holding the CRA accountable. After all, the notorious, chronic lack of consistency and transparency within the country's largest government department was no secret.

Even MP Gallant recognized that Bill C-462 would not resolve the inherent problems within the system, by affirming that, "The application process is still complex, and the tax credit is difficult to obtain." She had no choice but to recognize that not all companies assisting with the application and appeal process were preying on Canadians with disabilities.

Of course, I am not suggesting that all of these businesses deserve such hard criticism. This legislation is not directed toward legitimate tax practitioners who provide a valuable service. Make no mistake this bill is all about going after those whose intentions are not so honourable.

The only problem was the lack of credible evidence. Although these companies had been singularly targeted for their "predatory practices" there was no one to prosecute. Even so, the Act to restrict fees received royal assent on May 29, 2014.

In order to protect their own interests, eleven companies, representing hundreds of DTC consultants, and more than 200,000 Canadians with disabilities, banded together and formed the Association of Canadian

Disability Benefit Professionals, with its own code of conduct. On December 17, 2014, the Association met with senior officials of the CRA offering to work together with them, to establish a reasonable fee structure. But to no avail.

When Mr. Medjuck invited me to meet with him and his staff at the NBA offices in January 2016, I hesitated at first, since I was aware of the negative media reports of his early business practices. But it was an important opportunity to learn first-hand of the challenges dealing with the CRA from the experiences of 120 employees manning 1,600 calls a day. Mr. Medjuck reserved the Cambridge Suites in the downtown hub of Toronto for my stay. The irony didn't escape me when I discovered that the hotel was built by his uncle Ralph Medjuck. I had interviewed him back in 1980 for *Halifax* magazine, when we lived in Nova Scotia. As one of the top commercial builders in the city, he had his share of run-ins with government regulatory agencies.

I met with Katherine and Jason, two of the department heads at NBA, who were passionate about making a difference in the lives of disabled Canadians. They demonstrated an unwavering commitment to ensure that those eligible for the DTC were able to access the tax credit. They allowed me to examine dozens of files (with personal information carefully redacted) that were rejected by the CRA. The lack of competence by so-called "trained" government assessors was astounding. It was even more incomprehensible when the eligibility criteria was incorrectly applied and how long it took to have it fixed. Many of the rejections were simply form letters without addressing the medical evidence provided by health practitioners. Not surprisingly, the majority of rejected claims were overturned on appeal. Mr. Medjuck claimed that his success rate was 66 per cent.

Whatever concerns Ms. Gallant may have had about "unfair charges" by so-called promoters, there was no urgency to regulate the industry. Not as far as the CRA was concerned, when it shelved the *Act* for another five years. In the meantime, the industry that the CRA opposed so vehemently continued to flourish. As the Agency kept tightening its eligibility criteria, there was no shortage of clients retaining the services of companies with the expertise to navigate the difficult and burdensome process on their behalf.

The CRA was failing on other fronts as well. In his Fall 2017 Report, the Auditor General Michael Ferguson found that two out of three calls to the CRA's call centres, 29 million throughout the year, went unanswered, due to active call blocking by the Agency. Calls that were able to get through, received wrong answers 30 per cent of the time. Is it any wonder that Canadians have had a long history of being frustrated with an inept government department that could not get its act together?

Ordinary taxpayers were not the only ones who had every reason to be frustrated by a government department that couldn't deliver the goods. The CRA was given a "D" grade by the Canadian Federation of Independent Businesses. A survey found that its agents were providing incomplete or incorrect answers 40 per cent of the time. Who knows how many people, even small businesses, relying on CRA's call centres for information, were led astray, and later penalized for inadvertently filing an incorrect tax return?

Disrespect for the rule of law

Cracking down on tax cheats has always been a problem. When that was not going to be enough, the Honourable Bill Morneau, Minister of Finance, had a better idea. After delivering his first Liberal Budget in March 2016, he sat down for an interview with reporter Bill Curry of *The Globe and Mail*. The finance minister hoped for a possible windfall of $3 billion a year in savings that could be achieved by cutting back on a broad range of tax credits. That was the same year that there was almost a 50 per cent increase in the number of rejections for people markedly restricted in their mental functions, with a potential savings of $221 million.

The willful discrimination against people impaired in their mental functions was repugnant. There were no guarantees that individuals already receiving the tax credit for 5, 10, 20 and more years would

230

continue to qualify under the terms of the revised Form T2201. The CRA was dishonest, providing misleading information about the eligibility criteria in its application form and related documents, indicating that anything less than 90 per cent was insufficient to qualify for the DTC. Such a threshold made it virtually impossible for people living with a psychiatric or autism spectrum disorder to meet the uncompromising eligibility criteria. Many doctors, including psychiatrists and psychologists, were reluctant to complete the new form for their patients, even if they had previously received the DTC.

I was angry at the injustice faced by thousands of ordinary Canadians who did not have the financial means to hire a lawyer or the mental capacity to represent themselves in court. Early on in my advocacy work, I decided to assist others as much as possible with their claims without charging for my services. I was drawn back into the fray by a clear case of discrimination against a highly productive, award-winning graphic artist, who also lives with a debilitating mental illness. Certainly, Vincent van Gogh would fail the test, despite suffering from severe bouts of both mania and depression, during the last few years of his life, when he managed to produce more than 300 of his greatest works of art.

Marlene was 55 years old and an employee of the Ontario government for almost 30 years. Despite numerous hospitalizations due to her erratic mood disturbances, Marlene managed to hold onto a senior position in her department, due to flexible hours and extensive accommodations in the workplace. Although she had received the DTC from 1990, when first diagnosed with bipolar disorder, Marlene was denied the tax credit in 2015 during a routine reapplication process. The CRA disregarded the medical evidence provided by her physician, supporting her "bipolar disorder, type I, severe, rapid cycling diagnosis."

Marlene was ready to throw in the towel, when Peter Weissman called me at the 11th hour, asking for assistance with her appeal to the tax court. Facing an early January deadline, I spent much of my Christmas holidays, holed up in my home office working on her case.

As far as I was concerned, she met the rigorous test of being markedly restricted in her mental functions "all or substantially all of the time" as stated in the Notice of Appeal filed with the court:

Marlene is always vulnerable to unpredictable, volatile mood swings and erratic behaviour indicating that she is markedly restricted in her mental functions, all or substantially all of the time, even though the external signs and symptoms may be perceived to be intermittent... Marlene's myriad of mental health problems is such a marked departure from the normal range of mental functioning and accepted human behaviour that her impairment justifies the tax credit.

The lawyer representing the Crown agreed and the case was settled out of court. While Marlene was granted the tax credit for all future years, most individuals living with severe mental illness are required to reapply for the DTC, usually every three to five years.

The diabetic debacle

As incomprehensible as it may seem, the CRA committed another strategic blunder that would galvanize the disability community once again. Senior officials changed the rules. And then, they lied about it. The self-inflicted diabetic debacle became the catalyst that led to the reinstatement of the DAC.

CRA's errant ways worked to our advantage. It is hard, if not impossible, to understand how a government department would carry out yet another contemptible scheme, to deny the DTC to people who require life-sustaining therapy, in secret, without consultation or justification.

The heinous act may have gone undetected except for the actions of Shane Nercessian of True North Disability Services Ltd. He was tracking hundreds of unprecedented rejections of DTC claims from diabetic adults throughout the summer of 2017. Previously, close to 100 per cent of their claims for life-sustaining therapy were approved. Suddenly, without warning, virtually all their applications were denied, although there had not been any recent amendments to the *Income Tax Act*. On their 19th birthday, diabetic children were also at risk of losing both the DTC and the RDSP.

Mr. Nercessian contacted Lynne Gaucher, Manager of the Disability Programs Section, and asked for a second review of 100 files. The results were the same. When Kim Hanson, Executive Director of Federal Affairs for Diabetes Canada, attempted to investigate Mr. Nercessian's findings, she also hit a brick wall. During a radio interview she shared her frustrations, trying to determine where the breakdown was occurring, while CRA claimed, "There's been no change in policy."

The Honourable Diane Lebouthillier, Minister of National Revenue, repeatedly refused to admit to any wrong-doing in heated exchanges during Question Period in the House of Commons. She maintained that, "There has been no change to the eligibility criteria for the DTC related to diabetes. And the CRA has not changed its decision-making process with regard to the DTC."

There was no choice but to go public. Diabetes Canada along with JDRF (formally known as the Juvenile Diabetes Research Foundation), called a press conference on Sunday, October 22, and the evening CTV News reported their grievances:

Diabetes Canada was among the groups… to publicly denounce what they say is a claw back of a long-standing disability tax credit to help them manage a disease that can cost the average sufferer $15,000 annually… In recent months, the agency officials and Minister Lebouthillier have for the most part rebuffed their overtures.

Despite all the evidence to the contrary, the CRA continued with its false claims when interviewed by the media. On October 23, *Global News* reported that the CRA spokesperson, John Power, acknowledged that, "the concerns raised on Sunday are 'worrisome,' especially since the government has not changed the eligibility criteria for the credit, nor has the CRA changed how it decides who qualifies for the credit and who does not."

There was no acknowledgement of deception until a new firestorm erupted in the House of Commons.

Ms. Hanson had estimated that as many as 150,000 Canadians could lose their DTC and filed an ATIP request to determine whether the CRA had, indeed, implemented a major policy shift to reduce the number of diabetic claimants. And there it was, an internal memo sent to staff on May 2, 2017, stating, "We no longer believe that adults can possibly meet the requirement of 14 hours per week on their therapy." When she asked the CRA for the basis for such a false claim, there was no response. And yet, all adults, when required to reapply for the tax credit, were automatically excluded "unless there are exceptional circumstances... (or) the existence of other chronic conditions..." Of course, 14 hours was an arbitrary measure and did not reflect the severity or the costs associated with the monitoring and treatment of the disease.

When Ms. Hanson exposed the cover-up of an unjustified policy of presumptive denial to persons with diabetes, the CRA was backed into a wall. On December 8, 2017, *The Canadian Press* reported, "The Canada Revenue Agency took steps to quell a furor over what critics were calling its heartless treatment of diabetics." There was no choice for Minister Lebouthillier, but to reverse its controversial policy and review all of the applications for the DTC that had been previously denied.

Disability Advisory Committee

Any effort to fix the system was dependent on getting the DAC back on track. Maybe this time, we will get it right. In a joint letter to the Ministers of Finance and National Revenue dated April 12, 2016, Peter Weissman and I stressed the need to address serious problems with the administration of the DTC. We also co-founded the Disability Tax Fairness Alliance with representation from health charities and companies assisting people with their DTC applications and appeals.

When I was in Ottawa in early October 2017, I met with Minister Lebouthilier's Director of Policy, Anne Ellefsen-Gauthier. I provided her with a package of supporting reports and documents that I was handing out, while making my rounds in the capital on behalf of the Alliance. We were concerned about the spike in rejection of applications in all categories, where CRA assessors appeared to disregard the medical evidence, provided by health practitioners on behalf of their patients.

Ms. Ellefsen-Gauthier explained that the CRA had the right to question the integrity of the information provided by physicians. She shared her experiences as a lawyer representing the Quebec government when injured employees appealed decisions to deny their claims for compensation. According to her, not all doctors were providing an honest appraisal of their patients' injuries. As far as she was concerned, the ostensible reason for a doctor to endorse an ineligible claimant was to maintain a positive relationship with the patient. I was dismayed by her inference that doctors might overstate their patients' impairment to enable them to access the DTC. The CRA was shifting the blame for failed claims back to the medical profession, rather than accepting responsibility for its own shortcomings.

In the meantime, there would be no let-up of public indignation if steps were not taken to address the systemic problems in the administration of the DTC. So, I should not have been surprised to receive a call from Lynne Gaucher, who advised me that Minister Lebouthillier had approved the reinstatement of DAC and asked if I wished to be appointed to the new committee. It was a triumphant moment, another important personal victory. But the reality was far more sobering since it took such a humiliating fiasco to compel the government to act.

In an email from Ms. Ellefsen-Gauthier, I learned that the wheels had been set in motion to reinstate the DAC soon after the press conference exposed another dark chapter of government high-handed shenanigans.

Despite Peter's position as Co-Chair of the original DAC in 2005, not to mention his experience as a tax specialist for over 30 years, his offers to volunteer as a committee member went unanswered. I was bitterly disappointed that he was not invited to join the new DAC. No one in the tax business was more knowledgeable than Peter regarding the insurmountable problems accessing the DTC. As a person living with multiple sclerosis, Peter also understood the difficulties accessing the DTC, when the disease is characterized by unpredictable relapses followed by periods of remission.

Peter had been a staunch critic of new legislation on other tax matters introduced in 2017. Perhaps that was reason enough to reject him. Nevertheless, I was more than grateful to have Peter as a trusted advisor as I went head-to-head, once again, with a government not always willing to do the right thing because it cost too much.

The primary purpose of our committee was to improve access to the DTC. While we have succeeded to some degree, there hasn't been a whole lot to cheer about. Not that it was our fault. We had been through the wringer before.

There were five of us, veterans of the Technical Advisory Committee, established in 2003. Three of us were also members of the previous DAC created in 2005. It was both revealing and unnerving that we would be brought together, once more, to deal with many of the same administrative problems and discriminatory practices that we had grappled with before. Back then, we were all on the same page when the CRA and the Department of Finance refused to acknowledge the systemic divisiveness of their heavy-handed policies. Would we continue to support each other or would I need to dust off my boxing gloves, when meeting old and new adversaries in Ottawa?

I noted the irony in my journal:

Every day I am thankful for good health… and I pray to have the strength to keep fighting on behalf of people with disabilities… The reinstatement of the DAC is a huge, even giant step forward… we have rolled the rock back up the hill… now the real work begins.

The lack of progress on key issues was indicative of a bureaucracy violating basic principles of the *Income Tax Act* as well as disregarding case law that would test our resolve for the next three years. Our first annual report, *Enabling access to disability tax measures,* dealt at great length with the difficulties related to CRA's application of the 90 per cent threshold noting, "First it has no basis in law. Second, its use has been challenged by relevant jurisprudence."

None of that seemed to matter to senior officials, unwilling to accept our committee's recommendations. "There are many people being left behind," admitted Sherri Torjman, Vice-Chair of the DAC, during the press conference held on May 25, 2019, when we released our report. Dr. Cohen, Co-Chair of the DAC, provided the following explanation:

The 90 per cent interpretation is problematic for those with mental disorders and disorders that are characterized by episodic symptoms. Many people have symptoms less than 90 per cent of the time, but their condition is severe, prolonged and restricts them all the time. It is important that we clarify the eligibility criteria related to mental functions.

Two years later, we were still dealing with the same dogged determination by the CRA to thwart justice for thousands of children and adults with disabilities by blatantly disregarding the jurisprudence of numerous legal challenges, all the way up to the Supreme Court, in its interpretation of the legislation. During a virtual press conference when we released our second annual report, Dr. Cohen acknowledged that, "there are still significant legislative challenges remaining," noting our ongoing concerns regarding CRA's rigid interpretation of the "all or substantially all of the time" clause as being at least 90 per cent of the time.

When DAC released its third annual report on December 16, 2022, the 90 per cent threshold continued to be a matter of contention among its members. Nevertheless, the CRA has dug in its heels, and continues to apply a mathematical model rejected by the courts as an absolute determination of eligibility for the DTC.

Troubling testimony

I was back in Ottawa a week after the inaugural meeting of the DAC in January 2018, testifying before the Standing Senate Committee on Social Affairs, Science and Technology. The basis for the hearings was the difficulties accessing the DTC as well as issues related to the RDSP. The presentations from both sides could not have been more different.

The CRA refused to acknowledge the simple, but disturbing fact, that the eligibility criteria were being applied in a far more restrictive manner in recent years. As far as Minister Lebouthillier and senior officials of the CRA were concerned, their department had an exemplary track record of fair dealing, with more money than ever before being put into the hands of people with disabilities. It was a highly co-ordinated effort with everyone in agreement that all was well. Was there any doubt when Minister Lebouthillier's opening statement stressed the significance of empathy and transparency within her Agency?

Compassion and openness is all the more important when administering tax programs for our society's most vulnerable members, especially people living with mental and physical impairments.

Hundreds, if not thousands of Canadians, knew better. The violations of fairness and justice carried out with impunity by the Minister and her staff were legendary. So, it was hardly surprising that Senator Jim Munson, a former journalist and champion of families dealing with autism spectrum disorder, was blunt with his assessment of the alarming rate of rejections:

I still find it very upsetting. Your officials and others have heard the heart-breaking testimony before us. I still haven't figured out what happened inside the bureaucracy, what happened inside the ministry with all these rejections.... I can't quite figure that out... Everybody knows what's taking place and what's not taking place. They have been rejected by the hundreds, from what I understand.

Minister Lebouthillier countered with the same mantra that we have heard over and over again:

As I have said a little earlier, the eligibility criteria for receiving the DTC, the criteria haven't changed at all. They are exactly as they have been before. Neither has the Act changed. It's the same Act.

Clearly, Senator Munson was not satisfied with her dubious claim and said so.

You said nothing has changed. And yet, hundreds in the autism community have been turned down. We're dealing with a crisis in this community of autism. Something has happened. Something has taken place. I wish you would be a little more candid with us.

Of course, there had been changes. We all knew that. There was no question that the 90 per cent threshold was the essence of the problem facing Senator Munson and others advocating for fairness and justice. Dr. Cohen also testified that CRA's interpretation of the legislation was prejudicial toward a specific class of individuals, creating a "higher bar for persons with mental disorders to be deemed eligible for the DTC."

Senator Judith Seidman admitted that she was speechless. An epidemiologist and social services advisor, surely, she had heard plenty of shocking stories since her appointment to the Senate:

I shouldn't be speechless because I'm just so horrified and outraged listening to your presentations. The whole process, as we hear about it, from beginning to end, either is just obfuscation at best or, at worst, exploitative of the most vulnerable in our society.

I would like to start with a quote, Ms. Buchanan, from what you said, if I might. You said: 'In recent years, it's become evident that individuals, who previously qualified for the DTC for 10 years, 20 years and more are asked to reapply and then denied the tax credit on questionable grounds.' That's really astounding. What's the possible explanation for this? Is it that the CRA needs more tax monies, so they're just going after everyone they possibly can?

Senator Chantal Petitclerc, a wheelchair athlete and coach prior to her appointment to the Senate, was just as incensed:

It is outrageous and overwhelming to hear not only you but the witnesses before. The only thing that comes to mind is that it's really overwhelming when you think about all the concerns and issues and problems... It was always about the money... there was never any concern, that I am aware of, how many people are left behind.

I was personally disgusted by the cavalier attitude of each of the department's senior staff towing the same party line, asserting that all was well. The callous disregard of senior officials to the overwhelming mental and physical distress already expressed by so many, was reprehensible. Despite all the "heart-breaking testimony" of people who had lost thousands of dollars in tax relief and RDSP contributions, the federal government refused to accept responsibility for its shameful and deceptive practices. There was no recognition of the terrible anguish experienced by these individuals who lost important income supports though their medical condition remained unchanged.

Just as despicable was CRA's long standing policy deliberately withholding documents, such as questionnaires that doctors and others were asked to complete, when providing additional information to support a patient's claim. I had raised these concerns more than 15 years ago when I was a member of TAC, and subsequently advised that the information between the doctor and the CRA was confidential. It always seemed to me that such a violation of the taxpayer's rights, when objecting to a wrongful decision, was tantamount to an admission of guilt.

Not surprisingly, Ms. Nancy Chahwan, Deputy Commissioner of the CRA, denied any inappropriate activity by CRA assessors, stating: "We do not substitute our judgment for the medical practitioners." Her claim was echoed by Frank Vermaeten, Assistant Deputy Commissioner and Co-Chair of DAC. "Their job," he said, "is not to second-guess what the medical community has provided."

Contrary to polite assurances, their testimony was in stark contrast to an email from Lynne Gaucher, sent to me on September 8, 2017, claiming that, "The CRA has the duty to administer and enforce the *Income Tax Act*, and consequently has the authority to question the medical evidence provided by a medical practitioner." This was an extraordinarily contentious issue, considering that people were often charged by their doctors, sometimes hundreds of dollars, to complete the application form, as well as the follow-up questionnaire in many instances. And where was the justification to question a doctor's judgment? I had already testified at the Senate hearing that, "the CRA should not have the authority to disregard medical evidence certified by qualified health care practitioners acting in good faith... Unless there is clear evidence of fraud."

Health reporter André Picard also criticized CRA's shameless dismissal of the clinical findings by an applicant's doctor, in his opinion piece in *The Globe & Mail* on July 3, 2018: "When medical professionals provide a diagnosis – based on rigid criteria, no less – pencil pushers in the CRA have no business second-guessing a medical decision."

Senator Richard Neufeld, a former councillor, mayor, and Member of the Legislative Assembly of British Columbia from Fort Nelson, also questioned the overall decision-making process and whether there was a deliberate attempt to sabotage the efforts of people reapplying for the DTC:

I have certainly heard, from where I live in British Columbia, a lot of people complaining that all of a sudden, things have changed dramatically for them. So my question is, when I hear thousands of changes, some people have been on disability for five years... some even longer, all of a sudden, find themselves cut off. We had the minister here, she said nothing changed in the regulations, nothing changed in the legislation, nothing changed... (but) something changed. Maybe you can help me here. Were all of these (applicants) poorly adjudicated before? Or is it poorly adjudicated now when you start kicking them off? Something changed.

These people deserve an answer of some kind. How can you be on disability for five or eight years or longer and then, boom you're off? Something went wrong either prior to now because there is a spike. Everyone has admitted that. Or something is being done wrong now. Something changed!

Mr. Vermaeten had no choice but to concede that there was a major policy shift that affected diabetics, acknowledging that, "There certainly was an administrative change with unintended consequences." However, in a brazen attempt to pass the buck, he suggested that the medical community was looking for clarification of the eligibility criteria for people living with type 1 diabetes. That may be so. But surely, it was never the intention of doctors to make it more difficult for their patients to access the DTC. In an effort to demonstrate goodwill on the part of the CRA to fix the problem in an expeditious manner, Mr. Vermaeten attempted to cover up a deliberate tax grab with half-truths in his testimony:

Several months later, we did hear a lot of feedback that this (action) was increasing the rejection rate. And we, obviously, immediately, looked into this and we responded... and we have since corrected that action.

There was no apology.

Contrary to his testimony, there was never any urgency to resolve "unintended consequences." I was disappointed to hear Mr. Vermaeten so blithely steer clear of responsibility for creating such chaos in the lives of so many families. Instead, he concluded his testimony by further minimizing the devastating impact of hundreds of people unjustly denied the DTC when he said: "It was a very narrow range of applicants... it was a relatively small group."

By the time the CRA withdrew its controversial policy directive, 2,267 applicants had been denied the DTC. These individuals lost an important tax credit to help cover the cost of insulin therapy. Many would also lose their RDSP, along with government contributions made in the previous ten years. Such a "narrow range of applicants" represented over $3.4 million in tax savings for the government and millions more in bonds and grants clawed back from closed accounts.

Clearly, the Senate Committee was not buying the carefully orchestrated rhetoric from CRA senior officials. In its report, *Breaking Down Barriers: A critical analysis of the Disability Tax Credit and the Registered Disability Savings Plan*, issued in June 2018, Senators called on the government to implement a more "compassionate" application system for the DTC. The report also highlighted a 50 per cent increase in rejections in the mental functions category.

If Senators were looking for an explanation behind the spike in rejections in 2016/2017, it was not forthcoming. Neither Ms. Chahwan nor her colleagues had a clue and said so. That was the year top officials at the CRA were earning $6.9 million in bonuses, up to $35,000 each, based on annual salaries, many in the $200,000 range. Although she claimed that her staff was investigating the unusual, sudden increase in rejections, there was never any follow-up to Senator Munson's concerns.

When I was a member of DAC, I was also looking for answers. If I couldn't get at the truth, who could?

The CRA never addressed the emotional fall-out when someone had been rejected, regardless of his or her medical condition. Their suffering was of little or no consequence to senior staff of a government department, as long as it refused to acknowledge that a chronic and persistent mental illness was a real disability, within the scope of the legislation.

In an email from Brian, he underlined the importance of a sympathetic ear when confronting a government bureaucracy that routinely discriminates against people living with bipolar disorder. Although the symptoms may not always be present, the underlying condition affecting his well-being was challenging all of the time.

You are so kind Lembi it makes me want to cry... I really mean that... we are strangers but have so much in common... your empathy means so much to me... this is such a lonely illness... but you are right about my family... I adore all of them and for some reason they have all stuck with me... The problem is my mania makes me feel invincible, dismissive of everyone.

Consider what I did within the same three-month period of directing the account transfer (of funds). I impulsively decided and convinced my wife to sell our condo with no alternative living plans. Then I decided it would be a great idea to immediately travel through Italy for six weeks, again without addressing the living arrangements when we returned.

Half way through the trip, on my birthday, for whatever reason, I declared that I had healed myself and discarded all my meds. My wife said I became very aggressive and she was frightened. Thankfully I am a pacifist by nature so nothing violent, just reckless and stupid behaviour. After about ten days without meds, I was in really bad shape. When we returned, my wife immediately took me for help and I considered readmission. Anybody that can live with me deserves a special place in heaven and thank you kindly for all your gentle support.

Brian's application for the DTC was eventually approved, but it should never have been rejected in the first place. There was no basis for the CRA to be disrespectful when Senator Munson testified that hundreds of people living with autism had also been turned down without a valid reason. Otherwise, surely, there would have been a sense of urgency to resolve some of the "concerns over the administration of the DTC" outlined in the Senate report.

Instead, the government's formal response to the Senate Committee took eight months to draft and said little of substance. Some of it was downright hypocritical, with empty promises, such as "a dedicated telephone service where claimants for the DTC can call and get direct access to a specialized agent." The problem with administrative changes to provide greater support to Canadians claiming the DTC was the age-old excuse, that it cost too much.

The CRA has always relied on the Department of Finance for approval of amendments to the *Income Tax Act* associated with cost implications. There were no additional funds forthcoming following the Senate hearings, to ensure, at the very least, that the CRA was meeting its mandate of fair tax treatment of people who needed it the most. Certainly not from the man responsible for the public purse.

Finance Minister Morneau had more pressing matters to deal with throughout his term in office. Investigations into the personal affairs of the wealthy businessman revealed ethical violations, including a non-payment of $41,366 in luxury travel expenses to the WE Charity, after visiting its operations in Ecuador and Kenya in 2017. The public was incensed by his failure to disclose such a sizeable gift. Less than a month after admitting to his role in the charity scandal that rocked the Liberal government that summer, Minister Morneau handed in his resignation to Prime Minister Justin Trudeau on August 17, 2020.

The money heist

No action by the CRA was as ruthless and punitive as denying the DTC to young people living with autism, and clawing back government grants and bonds paid into their accounts. Is it any wonder that Senator Munson was on the verge of losing his cool during the Senate Committee hearings on the DTC and the RDSP?

Mike was unjustly denied the tax credit when asked to reapply for the benefit in 2016, which he had received from birth, that is, from 1990 to 2015. Incomprehensible as it may seem, his $60,000 RDSP account was at risk of being closed by the CRA and he would have lost tens of thousands of dollars in government contributions. Mike was a 27-year-old severely autistic and intellectually challenged young man, living with his mother in Edmonton, Alberta. Since 2009, Mike had held a part-time job with a major corporation, clearing and cleaning tables, and washing dishes in the employee cafeteria.

It did not take long to discover that the internal appeals process was a sham, when clear and irrefutable medical evidence, including extensive psychological reports, were simply ignored. The DTC was denied, according to the appeals officer, because Mike could now bathe himself and take care of other personal hygiene needs. When filing Mike's Notice of Appeal in tax court, I relied on the precedent-setting decision in my husband's case:

The facts clearly demonstrate that the Appellant is unable to perform the necessary mental tasks required to live and function independently and competently in everyday life. His myriad of mental challenges is such a marked departure from the normal range of mental functioning that his impairment justifies the tax credit.

Although Mike's case was quickly settled out of court, the CRA has not recognized that his mental impairment is permanent. He will be required to reapply for the DTC again in 2024 to continue to receive the government contributions for his RDSP.

In February 2019, I met with my MP, Murray Rankin in his Ottawa office, along with members of the NDP shadow cabinet, to stop the steal. I remember their expressions of indignation with a government policy that could be so downright nasty, considering the program was specifically set up to help disabled Canadians save for future needs.

Soon enough, persistent lobbying efforts from all sides paid off. The Budget tabled in the House of Commons on March 19, 2019, ensured that RDSP funds were safe when individuals were asked to reapply for the DTC. They could keep their accounts, including government bonds and grants, even if they no longer qualified for the tax credit.

Four years in Tibet

The heavy artillery was out on a conference call when I transgressed, apparently unfitting of a member of DAC. Seems that someone was offended when I responded in an "inappropriate manner" to a father's relentless pursuit of justice for his intellectually challenged daughter.

Robert had written to Prime Minister Trudeau, describing his odyssey as "Four Years in Tibet" due to the "interminable fumbling" by the CRA of his daughter's file. In his letter, Robert provided the details of his "lamentable journey" that stretched from May 2014 to December 2017 before Beatrice's DTC was reinstated.

In an email to the father, I suggested that he share his letter with our committee. I suspected that the reason to deny the DTC was the fact that Beatrice was capable of cleaning her own room despite severe limitations in many other areas. Apparently, that was reason enough for the CRA to cut her off and I said so, in my email, which somehow made its way up the ranks to senior staff.

No wonder, Robert was confused by the carefully crafted but nonsensical explanation from the CRA, citing Verse Number 82357 from its *Taxation Operations Manual* to disallow the DTC:

For this credit, difficulties in areas such as working, housekeeping, social or recreational activities, academic skills, managing a bank account and/or driving a vehicle are not considered marked restrictions in performing the mental functions necessary for everyday life.

Robert's persistence paid off. After several years of reviews and appeals, he managed to have his daughter's application evaluated by a registered nurse affiliated with CRA's Ottawa office who supported the claim. Not everyone, however, has the stamina to keep fighting, for years, if necessary, to achieve a just result.

Louise sent me an email when her son, burdened by the disordered thinking caused by schizophrenia, was denied the DTC although he had also been receiving it for many years: "I appreciate all you have done for us," she wrote, "but I am not prepared to fight this decision. I just don't have the will to put any more energy into this at this time." Louise was not alone, all the more reason for me to intercede to protect her son's access to the DTC and his RDSP.

John Adams, a former Toronto Councillor and Co-Chair of the Disability Tax Fairness Alliance also assisted individuals with their claims. He pulled no punches in an interview with *Blacklock's Reporter*, dated June 3, 2019, criticizing the CRA when it published the *Disability Tax Credit Promoters Restrictions Regulations* in the *Canada Gazette*, setting the maximum fee of $100 that anyone can charge, regardless of the work involved with the application process for the DTC:

I do pro bono work for a community with intellectual challenges, people who applied for the tax credit and were denied. My record is fifteen wins out of fifteen appeals to the Tax Court of Canada. These were all unjust denials of claims... Their letters of refusal are deliberate and maliciously misleading to the taxpayers... There are consultants out there who do an incredible job of helping these people.

And that was the problem.

The majority of people needing assistance with their applications had no choice but to rely on consultants who worked closely with them to ensure that they were accessing the income supports to which they were entitled. In the same interview, NBA's President, Akiva Medjuk claimed that, "There has been an ongoing process to give as few people as possible the Disability Tax Credit... We make the CRA look bad because we don't stop fighting, and (now) they are trying to shut us down. They are destroying an industry that actually helps people... Not a single company is able to operate under these Regulations."

Predatory practices

There was never any evidence of a widespread, grand rip-off scam by these companies, conspiring with their clients to cheat the tax system. If there had been illegal activity by nefarious schemers, the CRA should have stopped them in their tracks. Indeed, the Agency certainly had the means, the power, and the duty to do so. Instead, the CRA was allowing a false narrative to persist, always referring to these legitimate businesses as "promoters," suggesting (on its website) that, "they deliberately make false statements to assist their clients in tax cheating, all the while obtaining a financial benefit."

The CRA was well versed in its own predatory practices over the years, pulling one stunt after another. Some were sneaky and underhanded; others were shrewd and duplicitous. Each one may have been carefully calculated to limit access to the DTC.

None was as deceitful as the PowerPoint (PPT) presentation sent by Minister Lebouthillier's office in June 2017 to all MPs, ostensibly to clarify the eligibility criteria for the DTC. Unless they were familiar with the legislation, they would not have known that the PPT guideline, imposing an inflexible 90 per cent threshold to define "all or substantially all of the time," was at odds with the parliamentary and legislative intent of the *Income Tax Act*. Instead of being helpful, as far as enabling MPs to provide assistance to their constituents, the PPT guidelines represented a new low by a government determined to maintain strict controls on dollars allocated to the DTC program.

My MP Murray Rankin wasn't falling for a cheap trick designed to deceive all 338 elected representatives in the House of Commons. A law professor at the University of Victoria before entering politics, he agreed that the CRA had overstepped its mandate. In a rebuke of the false missive from Minister Lebouthillier's office, his terse message to her, in a letter dated June 30, 2017, emphasized that imposing the inflexible 90 per cent threshold in the PPT, "is not supported by your own policies nor the *Income Tax Act* nor Tax Court of Canada rulings."

The Minister's office was also being less than honest, when responding to an inquiry from the Conservative MP Alex Nuttall from Barrie, Ontario, by providing only the most extreme examples of disability in yet another effort to limit access to the DTC such as:

Feeding: whereby an individual needs feeding tubes at least 90 per cent of the time.

Speaking: whereby an individual must rely on other means of communication, such as sign language, at least 90 per cent of the time.

Hearing: whereby an individual must rely completely on lip reading or sign language at least 90 per cent of the time, to understand a spoken conversation, despite the use of hearing aids.

Eliminating: whereby the individual needs a device for eliminating which causes them to take an inordinate amount time to manage bowel or bladder functions.

I sent an email to Ms. Ellefsen-Gauthier expressing my shock to see that her boss had signed onto a document that was "just plain wrong." There was no response from her, or the Minister. If she couldn't get it right, was it any wonder that information from others under her watch was also suspect?

The sad truth was that the CRA could not be trusted to provide reliable tax advice. And there was no where else to go except companies with the resources to help people navigate an onerous and complex system, to claim not only much-needed tax relief, but also additional financial benefits. While MP Gallant may never have had any intention of punishing everyone, only the bad apples, the CRA appeared to be determined to wipe out the very industry that held it accountable.

And our committee was the perfect patsy.

Abuse of power

It may be a coincidence, even a stretch of my imagination, whether it was intentional or not, but the CRA managed to use our committee to do its dirty work. No doubt about it, we were duped.

The CRA was suggesting that limiting fees to a maximum of $100 was based on our recommendations. Nothing could be further from the truth. Some of us doubted that $100 would cover the work required for the simplest cases, let alone applications that were complex, requiring considerable time, with some taking years to resolve. Although our committee supported setting limits to the fees that these DTC consulting companies could charge, we recognized that a fixed rate was not appropriate in all cases. We discussed the need to strike a balance, ensuring that vulnerable populations are not financially disadvantaged, and at the same time, adequately compensating those that are helping them to get the benefits to which they are entitled. None of us contemplated the possibility that CRA would impose a flat fee, so low, that it could drive them out of business.

According to the Regulations, the fee, first introduced during consultations held in 2014, was based on an estimation of "an hour of work for professional tax services at $100 an hour." That was a bad joke back then. It soon became an offensive proposition, with CRA refusing to admit what was so obvious to everyone else, that the application process was hardly a simple matter. If it was such a walk in the park, why would 200,000 people use the services of DTC consultants and forfeit a percentage of their refund?

Without question, discussions of DTC consultants, the so-called "promoters," had always been very divisive during our meetings. But we were not about to cut off the very lifeline that so many people relied on. While we agreed that there was a need for regulations to protect individuals from being exploited, we never dreamed that the CRA might have had only one game plan in mind.

It soon became painfully clear, that the very industry, challenging the indiscriminate abuse of discretion by anonymous assessors in tax centres across the country, would self-destruct under the new regulations. My only question was whether the CRA was guilty of a con job, deliberately misleading our committee by initially assuring us that the $100 fee would only cover the costs related to the application process. And then, reversing its decision, without further consultation with our committee, deciding that the $100 fee would also include additional time spent filing an objection with the Appeals Division, if the applicant's claim was denied.

I was not only shocked but also utterly dismayed at CRA's violation of our trust. Surely abandoning the disabled, by limiting access to professional and legal advice, was not the intent of the MPs or Senators that supported Bill C-462.

Peter Weissman wrote about the dangers of abolishing our current system of checks and balances in an email to our committee:

By eliminating the ability of advisors (accountants, lawyers and DTC consultants) to provide assistance and advocacy, the CRA's power in this area is absolute. This is not how our tax system works given that the CRA is right all the time unless the taxpayer can prove them wrong. Under the model you are forcing on Canadians… you are not protecting the vulnerable, you are harming them. I know this is not the intention, but this is the reality.

However modest the $100 fee might sound, it could become a huge barrier for single mothers and seniors living close to the poverty line, that do not have extra cash on hand to wager against an uncertain outcome. Not when CRA is "systemically oppressive" towards the most disadvantaged members of our society, according to former taxpayers' Ombudsman Sherra Profit. The lawyer from Prince Edward Island had plenty to say about the need for fairness in her annual report released on June 17, 2020.

In a *National Post* interview published the following day, she acknowledged "multiple instances where CRA's bureaucracy was overly rigid and had significant communication issues with taxpayers… that can be particularly problematic for vulnerable populations who don't always have quick or timely access to some basic services."

No one was more knowledgeable about the problems vulnerable individuals faced when attempting to access benefits and services from the CRA than Sherri Torjman, former Vice-President of the Caledon Institute of Social Policy, and the current Vice-Chair of DAC. "We recognize how very difficult and complex the system is," she conceded in an interview with *Blacklock's Reporter*, dated April 12, 2021, referring to the high rejection rates of claims for the DTC.

It was the same story almost 20 years ago, with Ms. Torjman as Co-Chair of the Technical Advisory Committee, noting the concerns made by various disability groups regarding problems in the interpretation and application of the DTC in our report *Disability Tax Fairness.*

Perhaps it would have been more prudent for the government to examine why these consulting firms have been so successful, before trying to shut them down. But the CRA has never demonstrated any real interest in fair play. Not when senior staff dismissed my concerns regarding numerous rejected claims, supported by a wealth of extensive documentation of the disabling effects of mental impairments. By eliminating companies assisting taxpayers navigate a Kafkaesque bureaucratic process, the CRA would essentially have carte blanche to act as it wished.

Day of judgment

Shane Nerscessian was having none of that. He and his business partners Ameet Gajjar and Steve Black recognized the need for professional advice and founded the True North Disability Services Ltd. (TNDS) in Surrey, British Columbia, in 2014. Their company is a leader in the industry with an A+ rating with the Better Business Bureau, with dozens of testimonials posted on its website, as well as a loyal following on Google and Facebook. Their business model is dependent on a reasonable and agreed upon contingency fee of 20 per cent for its services, regardless of how much time is spent on a file to resolve administrative errors and make necessary adjustments. And there have always been plenty of those. On the other hand, the $100 fee cap, set to take effect on November 15, 2021, would quickly decimate their business, leaving hundreds of clients in the lurch.

Mr. Nercessian had invested too much in his company to let an incompetent and irresponsible government department take it all away from him. He had exposed the last scandal implicating Minister Lebouthillier, that denied the DTC to thousands of people living with type 1 diabetes, struggling to cover the cost of managing their blood sugar levels. Now, he would take on the CRA.

Mr. Nercessian sought to have the proposed Regulations declared constitutionally invalid, since the jurisdiction to regulate professional fees for tax-related services by accounting and legal firms usually belonged to the provinces. But first, he appealed to the Supreme Court of British Columbia, requesting an injunction against the CRA from imposing the controversial $100 cap on fees.

The Crown's case fell apart when the legal defence team admitted that there was no evidence, not a single document, to support its argument of excessive contingency fees as high as 40 per cent of the refund. That's not to say it never happened. But no one was ever charged for stiffing the disabled. While the Crown argued that the fee cap was intended to stop criminal activity, there had never been any evidence of illegal activity since the CRA raided the offices of J & J Canadian Grants Company in September 2010. Nor had there been any reports of fraud by health practitioners or service providers, since MP Gallant introduced Bill C-462 in April 2012.

During the two-day trial, the Crown tried to discredit my affidavit, ostensibly, because I was not an "expert" in this subject. Apparently, my record of filing successful appeals over two decades was not proof positive of CRA being "notorious for its poor administration of the DTC."

Justice Harry J. Slade granted the injunction against the CRA. As far as he was concerned, TNDS would suffer substantial and irreparable losses, if the maximum fee that it could charge its clients was $100. On the other hand, the government itself would not suffer any tangible harm. After all, the CRA waited more than five years before drafting the Regulations, "to prevent the ostensible 'evil' or protect the public from an 'injurious or undesirable effect.'"

The decision also stopped the CRA in its tracks from imposing strict fee limits to lawyers, accountants and anyone else assisting taxpayers when appealing a wrongful decision. In a radical reversal of its controversial decision, the Agency immediately amended its proposal by limiting the $100 fee to the application process. Of course, the government should have known better than to interfere with the rights of Canadians with disabilities to access legal advice, when unjustly denied the DTC.

The following year, Mr. Nercessian was back to court arguing that the federal government did not have jurisdiction to regulate fee structures for businesses incorporated under provincial law. He was also challenging the Regulations on the basis that such a low fee is a breach of his charter rights since it would severely limit, and quite possibly eliminate access, to any meaningful assistance in the application process by people with disabilities. Another favourable decision is critical for DTC consultants to maintain the status quo for thousands of Canadians with disabilities, who might otherwise be left out in the cold.

In the meantime, the CRA has expanded the eligibility criteria for the DTC to all people living with type 1 diabetes. This is excellent news for approximately 300,000 people in Canada that now qualify for the tax credit and related financial benefits. And yet, others living with profoundly disabling medical conditions, such as fibromyalgia, characterized by widespread musculoskeletal pain accompanied by chronic fatigue, deprived sleep and memory loss, continue to find it next to impossible to qualify for the tax credit.

As indicated before, when there are winners, it seems to be inevitable, that it is at someone else's expense. As incomprehensible as it may sound, the CRA has, once more, turned its back on some of the most vulnerable members of our society, by raising the bar even higher for people already "markedly restricted" in their mental functions. Major revisions in 2022 to Form T2201 have narrowed the eligibility for the DTC to those, only with a "very limited capacity" in any one of 28 examples related to various mental functions. On the other hand, there have been no changes to the assessment tools for people with physical impairments, allowing for a broader, more comprehensive range of severity and frequency to qualify for the tax credit. All I can add is that I have a very limited capacity as far as understanding the lengths that the CRA continues to go to make it increasingly difficult for people living with a severe mental illness to access the DTC.

Elaine Smith of Toronto was in for a rude shock when her son's psychiatrist refused to complete Form T2201 for Jack, who was diagnosed with paranoid schizophrenia when he was a teenager.

Although Jack has been receiving the tax credit for almost 30 years, he must continue to file a new application every five years to continue to receive RDSP contributions from the government. Jack lives in a supportive housing facility that provides services 24/7 for its residents as well as assistance with medication management and anti-psychotic injections every two weeks. Nevertheless, his psychiatrist did not believe that his patient was sufficiently disabled, at least 90 per cent of the time, to continue to qualify for the DTC.

How is it possible that Jack no longer meets the eligibility criteria for the DTC? His medical condition hasn't changed. His needs haven't changed. But the CRA continues to disregard the rule of law and basic principles of justice, to treat all persons equally and fairly, by creating harsher tests for people living with mental impairments than those with physical disabilities.

In the classic novel, *Alice's Adventures in Wonderland*, Lewis Carroll provides a satirical look at government bureaucracy when Alice is asked by the Queen of Hearts to play croquet. She complains, saying:

I don't think they play at all fairly... they don't seem to have any rules in particular, at least, if there are, nobody attends to them – and you've no idea how confusing it is."

Part VII

Love is the Gift that Keeps on Giving

Chapter Eleven – Life's lessons

Forever love

Looking back, I still wonder if I could have prevented the havoc that threatened to tear our family apart more often than I care to remember. It's taken all of this time, more than 50 years, with the luxury of hindsight, to accept Jim's illness and its impact on his behaviour and moods. I have always loved my husband, even during the darkest days and periods of unremitting distress when I have felt so alone. At times, it was difficult to accept the painful reality of an illness that threatened our relationship, including Jim's erratic behaviour, the verbal abuse when he had too much to drink. As much as I complained about periodic alcohol abuse, Jim was rarely drunk. I was always relieved when he simply passed out as soon as he lay down in bed, regardless, if he was fully clothed with his shoes still on. Surely, Jim was not alone as far as making insulting remarks to family members when he was intoxicated. And yet, his callous disregard for my feelings is what hurt the most. After all the years of caring for him, when he was not well, and bailing him out, when he ran out of money, I felt that I deserved better.

As a result, there were plenty of instances when I was ready to give up on Jim, if for no other reason, than to protect my own sanity. Even our children, Jonathan and Larissa suggested, more than once, that I pack my bags: "Mom, get a life of your own." And so, I did, unknown to them, pack my bags, more than once, if only in my mind. One day when Jim wasn't home, I put aside a small box of my favourite CDs and hid them in my closet, as I plotted my departure.

But it wasn't that simple. What if Jim was doing the best he could, considering that he had no say in the genetic loading of the dice and a family history of mental illness? I was not always able to recognize whether he was in control of any, or all the decisions he made during our marriage. But I knew, deep down inside, if I abandoned Jim, and anything happened to him, I would not be able to forgive myself.

261

Besides, I didn't have the courage to go it alone. And why should I apologize for that?

Instead, I learned the benefit of keeping a personal diary, investing every year in expensive, beautiful, leather-bound journals, as if my thoughts had value, as if I had something important to say, even if it was just to myself. Sometimes, I tried to understand the insanity around me, whenever Jim was hospitalized, especially during the early days of our relationship when I wrote:

I want so desperately to have some happiness but all I face is pain and frustration. I don't know what to dream for anymore... all of my dreams have been shattered. I realize that I am not as strong as I want to make out sometimes... what am I trying to prove anyway?

Other times, I just tried to console myself when I was in a funk. One day, I couldn't bear the shameful reality of my own making, wondering about certain scenarios too embarrassing to write about – so I won't. On another occasion, I asked myself, "Who is going to read this stuff anyway? Not me. I really don't intend to relive these difficult days."

Some days were worse than others. Once, I ended my entry with, "Should I have opened the window and jumped." A few years earlier, on December 31, 2000, I had written the following brief note in my journal: "I am not so sure I want to spend another year with Jim."

With my marriage as rocky as it was, I needed a major overhaul of my own personal needs and desires. So, I decided to take piano lessons again after a forty-year hiatus, in hopes of relieving some of the stress within our relationship. Regardless of my limited finances, I called the Royal Conservatory of Toronto and signed up for lessons. Now there was a challenge, trying to get my fingers working again, dutifully following the Hanon finger exercises for "The Virtuoso Pianist." At least Jim had the good sense to keep a tight lid on any negative comments while I was trying to breathe some life into *Romance* by Jean Sibelius. That, however, was not the case with my culinary pursuits, when he was spoiling for a fight.

Like the night Jim came home after I had gone to bed and left freshly baked bran muffins to cool on the kitchen counter.

"How long are the muffins going to stay out here?" he demanded.
"I'll put them away soon," I assured him. "Is anything wrong?
"It smells like a bakery here," he complained.
"What's wrong with it smelling like a bakery?"
"An apartment is not supposed to smell like a bakery."

What's wrong with him? I wondered. Surely, everyone else would love the aroma of fresh baked goods in their home.

Back then, I wrote almost every day. And now, almost not at all. Only the briefest notes have found their way onto the pages of the lovely *New Yorker Desk Diaries* that Santa leaves under the Christmas tree every year. But the memories help stitch the narrative together, how we managed to stay true to each other, when a precarious balance existed between sanity and madness. The belief that I was always Jim's true love has sustained me over the years.

Despite some very difficult periods during our relationship, I never doubted that Jim loved me unconditionally. That was evident when I faced yet another cancer scare a few years ago. Although the pathology was not nearly as serious as my previous medical diagnoses, I was devastated by the extent of the surgery for basal cell carcinoma with a long trail of stitches working their way along the length of my nose. I worried about the scarring; and the healing process took longer than I care to remember. But Jim was unfailing with his love and support, reminding me, that in his eyes, I was still beautiful.

Even as I aged, Jim never found fault with my looks. With such devotion and loyalty, how could I have left Jim when he wasn't well? Certainly not when he wasn't aware that he was ill, and under no circumstances when he was always compliant with his meds. While the effectiveness of psychotropic drugs was not absolute considering the severity of the disease, the meds allowed us to stay the course as Dr. Jamison notes in *An Unquiet Mind*:

263

No amount of love can cure madness or unblacken one's dark moods. Love can help, it can make the pain more tolerable, but, always, one is beholden to medication that may or may not always work and may or may not be bearable. Madness, on the other hand, most certainly can, and often does, kill love through its mistrustfulness, unrelenting pessimism, discontents, erratic behaviour, and, especially through its savage moods.

Thankfully, early on, Jim realized that he couldn't weather the extremes of manic highs and depressive lows. He never considered cruising at speeds in excess of 160 kilometers per hour, a risk while experiencing elevated moods. And the suicidal thoughts at the other end of the spectrum always brought his world to a standstill, leaving him despondent and fearful. Like a type 1 diabetic dependent on insulin, Jim is dependent on lithium and other medications to prevent dangerous mood swings caused when neurotransmitters, such as serotonin and dopamine in the brain, are out of sync.

The harmful legacy of the anti-psychiatry movement

Bipolar disorder is a deadly disease if left untreated. And yet, anti-psychiatry activists continue to reject advances in neuroscience as well as indisputable evidence of the efficacy of mood stabilizers and other drugs to treat the symptoms of severe mental illness.

In 1960, Thomas Szasz, an American psychiatrist and academic, published *The Myth of Mental Illness*, denying the existence of mental illness altogether. Dr. Szasz's book is still in print and continues to be required reading in some university and college sociology programs. In 1991, Peter Breggin, an American psychiatrist and student of Dr. Szasz, published *Toxic Psychiatry*, not only criticizing the biological model of mental illness, but also labelling psychotropic drugs as "the worst plague of brain damage in medical history."

In 2016, the late Bonnie Burstow, a senior lecturer at Ontario Institute for Studies in Education at the University of Toronto, created a firestorm of controversy when she launched a scholarship in her name for a thesis student conducting related research supporting her anti-psychiatry beliefs.

However, no individual or organization has fuelled the anti-psychiatry movement more aggressively than the Church of Scientology. By recruiting celebrities such as John Travolta and Tom Cruise, Scientologists have raised enormous financial resources to support its agenda. In December 2005, influential public officials and entertainment industry leaders gathered in Los Angeles to mark the opening of its new museum, Psychiatry: An Industry of Death.

Just as distressing are some of the claims made by leading voices on mental health and addictions, denying the genetic basis for bipolar disorder, including Canadian physician and author, Dr. Gabor Maté. In his new book *The Myth of Normal*, co-authored with his son Daniel Maté, he refutes the biological approach to mental illness, when he writes about the "faulty assumptions that exemplify the simplistic genetic narrative."

When scholars, educators, doctors, nurses, politicians and religious institutions brush off the disabling effects of a mental illness as a personal weakness or moral failure, or the manifestation of early childhood trauma, is it any mystery that Jim has had to fight in the courts for financial benefits routinely granted to people living with physical impairments?

I have never understood the invasive culture of deception, year after year, since 1992, when the Department of National Revenue first acknowledged problems with the determination of eligibility for the DTC. And yet, there was no action to counteract the criticism that the restrictive guidelines prevented eligible applicants with a severe disability from accessing the tax credit. Over the years, hundreds of thousands of people have been denied the DTC. It is anyone's guess, how many legitimate claims have gone by the wayside, with no one to pick up the pieces.

In order to assist as many people as possible, I posted a new website www.fightingforfairness.ca online, providing them, as well as health practitioners, with the tools they needed to navigate the review and appeal process. I supported individuals who were denied the DTC without a valid reason by civil servants with insufficient medical and legal training to provide the "accurate, clear and timely information" regarding their decisions as required by the Taxpayer Bill of Rights.

I also took on other advocacy work, consulting for mental health charities, as well as lobbying for better access to psychiatric medications and treatment. I wrote several reports, developed policy guidelines, and created publications to assist organizations with their lobbying efforts. It was all about making a difference.

As supportive as Jim was, he was also keenly aware that my advocacy work was starting to take its toll. So, he decided to take matters into his own hands.

The gift that keeps on giving

As 2010 drew to a close, I noted in my journal: "It's been the very best Christmas..." I was quite overwhelmed with Jim's gift of a top-quality Nikon camera since I had never considered reviving a professional career in photography after leaving Elliot Lake more than ten years ago. Jim took care of that as well, by enrolling me in a course in stock photography. Since then, I have been selling my travel photos online to various media outlets throughout the world.

Is it any wonder that I have always been dependent on Jim's support? Right from the beginning, in the early days of our relationship, Jim restored my sense of self confidence when he encouraged me to pursue a career as a writer and photographer. Throughout our marriage, I would rely on Jim, trusting his incredible insight and uncanny vision, even now, as I struggle to complete this memoir, trying to capture the very essence of our relationship and why it has survived more than half a century.

Long before my 65th birthday, I suggested to Jim that it would nice to celebrate such a milestone in Paris. After all, weren't we still lovers? A master of maximizing the benefits of loyalty points, Jim booked us at the historic Le Grand Hotel in the heart of Paris. Our room had a magnificent view of Opera Garnier, the setting for the musical *The Phantom of the Opera*. When I stepped onto the narrow, wrought iron balcony, I could see the Eiffel Tower in the distance. There were other ways to save money, such as lining up for bus transportation from Charles de Gaulle Airport, which dropped us off in the public square across the street from our hotel.

Jim took charge of all the dinner reservations, including L'Atelier de Joël on my birthday. He wasn't taking any chances as far as securing a reservation at one of the top restaurants in the city, by booking online eight months prior to the date. In his email, Jim noted that the dinner would be a surprise to celebrate my birthday. The food was extraordinary and I have yet to manage to duplicate the creamy, buttery mashed potatoes served with the succulent rack of lamb. When the staff placed an elegant torte in front of me, with all of them singing *Joyeux anniversaire* I fell in love with Jim all over again.

As much as we enjoyed visiting the Louvre and other historic sites during the day, our most memorable experiences were in the evening as we dined at some of the best restaurants and cafes in Paris. Even travel writer and backpacker Rick Steeves embraced "a long, drawn-out 'splurge meal' as a wonderful investment in time and money" describing French cuisine "as sightseeing for your taste buds... as rich as visiting an art gallery."

The legendary 400-year-old La Tour d'Argent fit the bill perfectly. The lower floor is a museum of treasures and paintings collected over the years. A small elevator takes guests to the restaurant on the top floor with its stunning view of the Seine and the Notre Dame. Jim requested the wine list, a 400-page tome as massive as the Gutenberg Bible and then solicited the assistance of the sommelier for an appropriate pairing with the specialty of the house *canard à la presse*. Our tab included a picture postcard of a historic painting of the ritual carving of a duck, stamped with, *Le numéro de votre Canard: 1,099,478.*

Jim's attentiveness to details to ensure a wonderful evening has always been nothing short of astonishing. When we celebrated an anniversary lunch at Tulio, in Seattle, there were two, long-stemmed red roses at our table. Sometimes, it was just a glass of sparkling wine soon after sitting down for a dinner, when Jim had advised the restaurant that we were celebrating a birthday. A memorable meal at the legendary Charlie Trotter's in Chicago was followed by a tour of the kitchen and wine cellar by the late owner/chef himself, with a photo of the three of us, that hangs beside the shelving unit for our own pots and pans. More than anyone else that I had dated in the past, Jim understood the importance of intimate romantic dinners to rekindle the flame. It was also an excuse to dress up, and savour the luxury of just being with each other, holding hands across the table and still crazy in love.

Granted, there were extravagances that left me breathless, whenever I found a crumpled credit card receipt among Jim's papers. And yet, it wasn't as if I could have steered us to a more affordable restaurant, since I never knew, for the most part, where we were dining until we arrived at our destination. That was Jim. He was always very pleased with himself when he was able to surprise me. And why would I question Jim's mood when he was happy, even indulgent? Sure, there were occasions, when I felt guilty about not feeling guilty, as Jim catered to my weaknesses. As much as Jim's unbridled hypomanic behaviour may have threatened our marriage, paradoxically, and most importantly, it also kept the romance alive.

Like so many couples, we also have our song, "Send in the Clowns" from Stephen Sondheim's musical, *A Little Night Music* that opened on Broadway in February 1973, soon after we met. Somehow, we felt that the words reflected our relationship, full of bliss, after surviving rejection and loss of a previous relationship. As fate would have it, we found each other, and as we grew older, our love for each other sustained us. Despite the distractions over the years that upended our lives, and that of our children, there was always our song, that would restore the passion and intimacy so critical in our relationship.

Strength of character

We moved to Victoria, BC in 2009, escaping the long, bitterly cold winters of Toronto. Our new home was ideal for us, a spacious, two-bedroom apartment overlooking beautiful gardens with a fountain, waterfalls and a duck pond out back. Our son, Jonathan already lived in Tsawwassen on the mainland with his wife and two children. Our daughter Larissa and her family also moved to Victoria the following year, from Saint John, New Brunswick. The love we all shared for each other was absolute, as we supported each other, even during the most difficult days.

Our lives were forever changed on the fateful afternoon in May 2018 when Jim went out for a daily walk and ended up in the trauma unit of Victoria General Hospital. On his way home, while crossing at a well-marked crosswalk in front of our apartment complex, Jim was hit by a speeding pick-up truck, thrown onto the hood of the vehicle and then, onto the pavement. Despite broken bones and fractured ribs, he survived his physical injuries. However, symptoms of severe PTSD set in, soon after he came home from the hospital.

I was exhausted not only dealing with Jim's inability to care for his basic needs, because of the physical injuries, but also the disabling effects of PTSD. The presence of bipolar disorder complicated his recovery, exacerbating his fears, as he became increasingly anxious about leaving the apartment. Long after his physical injuries healed, Jim was still unable to tolerate the noise of traffic. He simply stopped venturing out on his own, except for medical appointments and kinesiology sessions.

According to a CRA appeals officer, the majority of PTSD cases "do not rise to the level of eligibility… because the impairment is episodic in nature." That is why far too many Canadian veterans find themselves in battle mode when forced to fight, on yet another front for their benefits.

Kevin served under retired Lieutenant-General Roméo Dallaire, where he was a witness of the horrific genocide in Rwanda in 1994 that left him permanently traumatized by the crimes against humanity. Notwithstanding the carefully scripted medical evidence provided by his doctor, Kevin received a form letter denying his application because the CRA assessor determined that the trauma he suffers from did not meet the 90 per cent threshold. There was no excuse for such blatant disregard for the doctor's evaluation of his patient when Kevin described his own unremitting pain in the following manner: "There are the times, I wish I could forget what I remember, and other times, I can't remember what I have forgotten." For them, the nightmares never end. Ask Lieutenant-General Dallaire, who still takes medications each day to relieve the symptoms of PTSD.

We are left with a sense of injustice wielded by a government that has lost its soul and crushed any dignity left when war veterans must struggle against all odds on the home front. Has it been a pernicious scheme all along to deny an entire class of people living with a serious mental illness the tax benefit designed to ease their financial burdens? I have no idea. In any case, I have never been able to understand the outright discrimination, for people like Jim, Kevin, and so many others, surely, just as deserving of our compassion as people with physical impairments. Where is the moral outrage and political will to do more to protect the rights of these individuals already stigmatized, labelled, shamed, judged, and held in contempt?

There are no easy answers. Otherwise, we would have resolved these injustices long ago. My best guess is that their strength of character gets in the way of a more conventional understanding of the disabling effects of a mental disorder. Jim has always been high functioning, smart and resourceful. That doesn't mean that his condition is any less severe. In *Buchanan v. The Queen*, Judge Campbell stated that Jim's psychiatrist was wrong to advise his patients "that this disability tax credit is intended for persons who are disabled to the point that they need almost continuous supervision and cannot even function in the home let alone the work force."

270

Being strong means accepting our destinies rather than running away from them. Being strong also means accepting the support from so many sources that enabled us to overcome some of the darkness. Remarkably, Jim has survived numerous hospitalizations, both voluntary and involuntary, as well as physical and chemical restraints, including harsh neuroleptic drugs and ECT. Jim also forged a successful career in public relations, although he was never well enough, long enough, to graduate from high school, let alone college.

When Jim encouraged me to write this memoir, he expected me to be completely honest about many of the challenges we have faced throughout our marriage. He wants others to have a better insight into the complexities of bipolar disorder and its impact on families and friends. Not everyone understands the risks, certainly not the threat of suicide or accidental death for one-third of the population. Then, there is the skewed decision-making process that is impossible for any of us to understand, including Jim. In the face of so many missteps along the way, he wants others to understand the importance of unconditional love that restores our faith in humanity and gives us hope for better days ahead.

I would not be honest, if I said all is well, when we continue to face new challenges, even as they exacerbate old wounds. But now, we share a much deeper meaning of love than when we first met. The euphoria of forever love is tamer, but all the more precious, since it has survived countless assaults over the years. Jim said it best in an anniversary card dated December 1, 1998:

We do not always agree and
our approach to life is somewhat different
yet the chemistry has always been there
and always will be.

Much love, Jim

Acknowledgements

My deepest thanks to my husband Jim who supported my decision to write about the challenges that we have faced over the years, not only fighting an unforgiving illness that threatened to draw us apart, time and time again, but also fighting for fair tax treatment for all Canadians with disabilities. And then, there are our children, Jonathan and Larissa who always stood by us, never judging, but always providing much needed love and support, especially when we needed it the most.

I would like to thank my good friends Robert Currer and his partner Dennis Pfohl who created the websites that have supported my advocacy efforts over the years. They have also played a most important role as far as ensuring that my memoir reaches readers such as yourself. I wish to thank Patricia DeWit for her wonderful cover illustration that tells my story so well, by capturing the sense of determination and urgency I felt each time I went to Ottawa to advocate on behalf of others.

I owe a special debt of gratitude to Marvin Ross who provided the assistance I needed to get this memoir into print and to Brenda Hillebrand and Marion Gibson who assisted with the proof reading of my manuscript. My gratitude also extends to many friends, including Melissa and Jerry McKee, Arlaine Bertrand, and others who read several drafts of the manuscript for their helpful advice. There is a special place in my heart to the individuals and families who have allowed their stories to be told, though some of their names have been changed to protect their privacy. Unfortunately, the stigma of mental illness continues to be pervasive in our society.

Over the years, there have been numerous individuals within the Department of National Revenue who have supported my efforts; several have been willing to review so-called "obvious" cases, and allow the DTC without the need to appeal many of them to the Tax Court of Canada.

I also wish to acknowledge Dr. Robert Cooke, who always provided excellent care for Jim. Unfortunately, he was caught in the conundrum in the interpretation of legislation that clearly discriminated against the mentally ill, who were not considered to be as disabled in their everyday lives as those with physical impairments.

I hope that my memoir encourages others to speak more openly about the challenges facing people living with a severe and chronic mental illness. While everyone is different, they all need our love, compassion and support. They also need the steadfastness of a government that recognizes that they too, are worthy citizens, and entitled to the same income supports as people living with physical impairments.

Appendix

Prime Ministers of Canada

Liberal – Jean Chrétien – November 4, 1993 to December 11, 2003
Liberal – Paul Martin – December 12, 2003 to February 5, 2006
Conservative – Stephen Harper - February 6, 2006 to November 3, 2015
Liberal – Justin Trudeau - November 4, 2015 to present

Committees

Technical Advisory Committee on the Status of Persons with Disabilities - April 2003 to December 2004

Disability Advisory Committee - July 2005 to February 2006

Disability Advisory Committee - January 2018 to present

Court cases

Buchanan v. Prudential Insurance Company of America 1992 - Ontario Superior Court of Justice

Buchanan v. The Queen 2000 - Tax Court of Canada

Attorney General v. Buchanan 2002 – Federal Court of Appeal

Hearings

Sub-Committee on the Status of Persons with Disabilities - November 20, 2001 to February 5, 2002

House of Commons debate regarding the need to overhaul the DTC - November 19, 2002

Standing Senate Committee on National Finance on Bill C-462 to restrict fees for companies assisting individuals with the Disability Tax Credit applications and appeals - April 1, 2014

Standing Senate Committee on Social Affairs, Science and Technology regarding the Disability Tax Credit and the Registered Disability Savings Plan – February 1, 7 and 8, 2018

Revisions to Form T2201 Disability Tax Credit Certificate

1996   Check boxes replaced narrative sections for diagnosis and description of the effects of the physical or mental impairment.

2000   Life-sustaining therapy added to include people living with cystic fibrosis and type 1 diabetes.

2005   Category of "Mental functions for everyday life" reflects amendments to the *Income Tax Act*. Category of "Cumulative effect" added to include people living with two or more significant restrictions caused by their physical and/or mental impairments.

2012   Introduction of the rigid 90 per cent threshold to define "all or substantially all of the time."

2021   Introduction of electronic Form T2201 with severity and frequency scales as a guide to describe an individual's limitations in a physical or mental impairment.

2022   Form T2201 includes amendments to the *Income Tax Act* for the category "Mental functions for everyday life." The severity and frequency scales are replaced with a more restrictive check list allowing the DTC only for individuals with a "very limited capacity" in a comprehensive list of mental functions.

Reports

2001   *The Current Disability Tax Credit Certificate, Form T2201, its Impact on Individuals with Disabilities and Case Law* – Lembi Buchanan

2002   *Getting it Right for Canadians: The Disability Tax Credit* – Subcommittee on the Status of Persons with Disabilities

2004   *Disability Tax Fairness* – Technical Advisory Committee on the Status of Persons with Disabilities

2018   *Breaking Down Barriers: A Critical Analysis of the Disability Tax Credit and the Registered Disability Savings Plan* - Standing Senate Committee on Social Affairs, Science and Technology

2019   *Enabling access to disability tax measures* – Disability Advisory Committee

CPSIA information can be obtained
at www.ICGtesting.com
Printed in the USA
LVHW080523170623
749596LV00002B/2

9 781738 947621